SO YOU WANT TO BE A NURSE

CHRIS DAVIES CURTIS

OTHER PUBLICATIONS BY CHRIS DAVIES CURTIS

Memoirs
So You want to Live on Sark
So You returned to Sark
From a Feudal Isle to Aotearoa
From Queen's Nurse to Godzone
To Sark and Beyond

Historical
Exits and entrances

Fantasy
The Healing Hands

Romances
Nurses in Training
Nurses at Large
Nurses in New Zealand
Nurses in Retirement
The Pledge
Escape to Sark
Ellie's Story

Copyright © 2023 CHRISTINE ELIZABETH DAVIES CURTIS

No part of this publication may be reproduced, stored in a retrieval system or transmitted in any form or by any means, electronic, mechanical, photocopying, recording or otherwise, without the permission of the author in writing.

Published by Chrisdaviescurtisbooks.com

Cover design by Bev Robitai
photoshop@xtra.co.nz

ISBN 978-0-473-66886-0

DEDICATION
To all nurses everywhere

INTRODUCTION

The pain in my right lower side had been going on for months but when I suggested it might be a 'grumbling appendix' the doctors smiled and muttered something about 'once a nurse always a nurse; we don't call it that these days.' They did finally agree to arrange a scan, fixed for a few days after I returned from my holiday in Australia.
Which probably saved my life.
The pain increased and I was not at all well, so was happy to return to New Zealand and relieved to keep my appointment. Within a few hours I was admitted to hospital with a mass in my abdomen, which proved to be an infected and leaking appendix. A week of intravenous antibiotics was prescribed, and I found myself a patient in a modern hospital with nothing much to do except observe the nurses and ward routine. It was all so different from my introduction to the profession over forty years previously.

******

PART 1
THE STUDENT
1958~1960

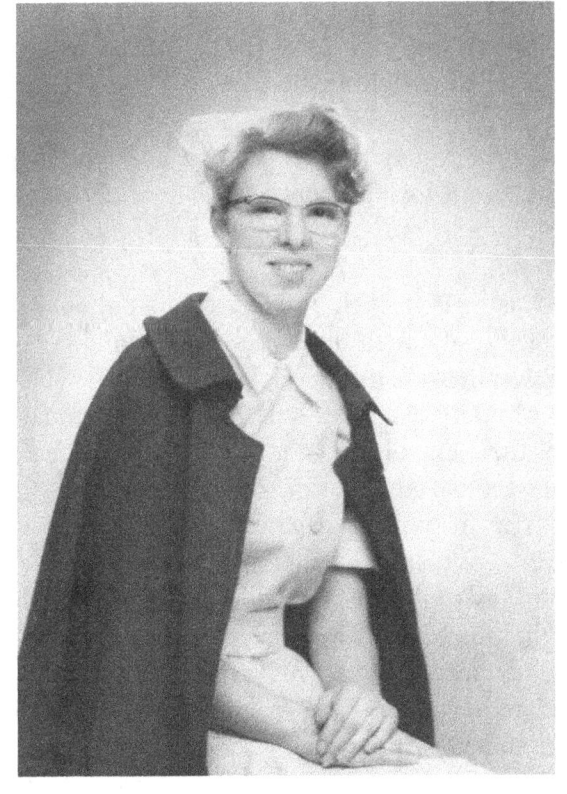

Student Nurse

1

I looked around the Hospital Chapel at the eighty or so other trainee nurses, wearing as I was, buttercup yellow dresses with soft white collars, short, cuffed sleeves and double-breasted buttoned fronts. I nervously reached behind to check no stray wisps of hair had escaped from the back of my starched cap. We had just been told this was important. There were so many things for us to remember; the newest student nurses just starting our training at the Queen Elizabeth School of Nursing, in Birmingham, England.

I watched the tiny motes of dust spiralling in a shaft of winter sunlight like a promise for the future, as I repeated the words of the Nightingale Pledge; *'I solemnly pledge myself before God and in the presence of this assembly, to pass my life in purity and to practice my profession faithfully. I will abstain from whatever is deleterious and mischievous and will not take or knowingly administer any harmful drug.'*

This was it: I was just eighteen years old, and the year was 1958. For the next three months I would be studying in the Preliminary Training school, and then if I passed the first of many examinations, I would become a trainee nurse for the General Register of State Registered Nurses. I did not realise at the time I had taken the first step towards over forty years as a nurse.

As we were dismissed by the Matron, we were told to make our way to the study block of buildings on the other side of the quadrangle. Fine needle-sharp pellets of sleet hit my face and smudged my glasses, as I wrapped the blue and red woollen cape around me. I ran across the concrete and was grateful for the strong brown lace-up shoes, trying to avoid the swirling dried leaves and patches of ice. As we arrived giggling and out of breath, we were brought up sharply by the strident voice of the grey clad diminutive figure of a Sister Tutor.

'Nurses; Nurses! Rule one; you do not run and must at all times maintain your dignity! Remember what you have just pledged. Now follow me into the classroom.' This was my introduction to Sister Murphy, who was to be our main tutor for the three months of preliminary training and the periodic study blocks we were to attend throughout the next three years. For the first months we were instructed in every technique from bandaging, giving injections, sterilising instruments, making beds, basic anatomy and physiology, hygiene and even the finer points of cleaning.

First, we were given instructions which made me feel I was back at school, or in a military barracks. 'Now, you will be here at Preliminary Training for three months. Each week you will have a day on the ward which you will be assigned to after the training. You will first have to sit a small examination.'

Sister Murphy paused and swept her steely gaze among us. 'Some of you will not get any further than that'

There was a general gasp as we were all now attentive.

'Yes, I know some of you have always wanted to be nurses; some misguided idea that you will be an angel of mercy.' There was a grim smile on the pinched features of the Sister. 'Well, think again! You have three years of hard labour, sleepless nights, exhaustion, and examinations and then, and only then, you may call yourselves nurses.'

I stole a look at the girls standing near me. The expressions varied from defiance, sulkiness, near tears and some like me, showed a resolution to succeed. 'Well, I'm not giving in,' I muttered. 'What else would I do? Teach? That was the only other alternative; anyway, I want to travel.' I had decided to join the Queen Alexandra's Royal Army Nursing Corps with a commission as soon as I was a State Registered Nurse. I was not one of those girls who had always wanted to be a nurse. At one time I had thought of trying for an art school, but I knew I was not good enough to make a living; I would have ended up teaching, which was the last thing I wanted to do. At my Grammar school there were not many alternatives offered. Teaching and nursing were the accepted professions unless you were bright and wealthy enough to go to university. Anyway, you were expected to get married and look after your husband and family as soon as 'Mr Right' came along. Nursing was regarded as an ideal training for that. 'Well not me' I had vowed, 'I want to do more with my life than that.'

'So now you can all go over to the notice board and check which bedrooms you are sharing. But first ...' again the steely gaze swept through our assembled group. 'A word of warning: absolutely no men allowed in the nurses home,' there was a subdued titter from one side of the room, which abruptly stopped as Sister swung to glare in that direction.

'You are allowed one late pass a month; otherwise you must be in by 10 pm. The doors are locked at that time and woe betide anyone who transgresses these rules.'

Feeling a little stunned I followed the others to look for my name and room number which I would be allocated in the Nurses' Home. I had always had my own room as had my only brother and was not happy about sharing. I determined as soon as I could I would live out, which would be in the second year. For now, I would have to share with at least one other nurse.

Patsy was a pleasant surprise: fun-loving and clever. I had always been a 'plodder,' having to study hard to gain my nine passes in the General Certificate of Education, not like my brilliant brother David who had just gained a place in a Cambridge University college. He had always been successful at his Grammar school in Stratford on Avon, where we grew up. His nose was always stuck in a book, even when we were taken for our 'family walks' our parents had insisted on.

My roommate and I could not have been more different, but I suppose my serious nature, spectacles and scraped back unattractively straight hair were a perfect foil for her vivacious attractiveness: at least I was no competition. It took me some time to become used to other girls popping in and out of our room; borrowing my best clothes and seldom returning them, but I had always been a little shy and enjoyed the company.

The three months of 'Prelim' as we learned to call this stage of our study, passed quite quickly. The hours we worked were similar to those recently left behind in our school years. Up at 7.30am and breakfast, followed by a short service in the Chapel. Then we were required to clean our rooms, the public area, and the toilets.

'I didn't expect to be a skivvy,' Patsy complained once to me, and I replied that I knew we were supposed to clean some places in the wards when we finally started the real nursing.

'I suppose it is to teach us that no jobs are too menial.' I added I had been told by a more senior nurse we had to do this sort of thing before a 'Matron's Round.' Patsy laughed: 'Yes I have heard that is like the Queen visiting; everyone on best behaviour.'

After the cleaning, lessons began in earnest, from 9am to 5pm, with a break of an hour for lunch. There were many lectures and then practical lessons to show we had been listening. I had thought myself reasonably dextrous but learning all the intricate bandages was a different story altogether. The worst were the 'Spikas,' as the figure of eight extensive bandage to cover a shoulder or even the back of a patient's neck, were called. The Sister Tutor often became exasperated with us as we disintegrated into giggles, when a volunteered 'patient' ended up looking more like an Egyptian mummy.

We even had instructions in such seemingly medieval practices as applying leeches and cupping. Being a country girl and with a keen gardener mother, I had become used to snails and slugs, but handling the slimy leeches even made me cringe, with visions of people wading through Amazonian wetlands, having to touch them with a lighted cigarette or salt to remove them.

'You may think these ways of medical care are archaic,' the Sister Tutor explained,' but some of you may find yourselves in less up to date facilities as at these hospitals. 'Leeches can draw haematomas...blood clots...from delicate areas and reduce infection, as they secrete peptides and proteins which work to prevent blood clots.' She went on to explain the process of 'cupping' which seemed easier to understand. 'Cupping therapy is an ancient form of medicine in which a therapist first heats the air inside the special cup then puts them on the skin for a few minutes to create suction. It is done for many purposes, including to help with pain, inflammation and to increase blood flow.'

I think Sister Murphy must have been a good tutor, for I remembered many things she taught us, years afterwards. She insisted on our smelling many different medicines and potions so we could recognise them and encouraged us to practice certain treatments on each other. Injections were first learned on an orange, and then later into another's' skin, using sterile water. One tip I used ever after, was to rub the site hard where the needle was to be inserted, and then tickle the place below while administering the injection. It seemed to take away some of the discomfort.

Although we chafed a little from the feeling of still being at school, the one day a week we had to work on a 'real' ward left most of us exhausted. 'How on earth will we cope when we have to work full time?' we moaned to each other, but it was soon time to become 'proper nurses.'

After a week's holiday we each returned to the ward we had been on during the Preliminary training.

2

I spent my week's holiday in Stratford on Avon with my parents. My father was the Customs and Excise officer there, and as a schoolgirl I had enjoyed travelling around to the outlying countryside with him. After the intense three months of study, I was happy to revert to my earlier habits and now Spring was beginning I enjoyed the lovely Cotswold orchards and villages.

For the first time in my life the seasons had changed without my noticing it. Always a country girl at heart I had been frustrated at missing my favourite time of the year, cooped up in the hospital environment. Already the blackthorn was in flower looking like sparkling frost on the dark brown twigs. Daffodils danced in the breeze and primroses and violets hugged the verges. The warm sandstone cottages with their pretty gardens were a world away from the cold green and cream corridors and wards I was soon returning to, and my father sensed my despondency.

'You don't have to do this, Chrissie...' I had always been his special girl... 'You'll find a nice young man I am sure and settle down.' If I needed any encouragement to continue my training, that was it.

'It will be better when I am on the wards.'

I was first allocated to a women's medical ward in the older General hospital. Our PTS group (Preliminary Training Student group number 206) had been split between the older General Hospital in the centre of the city, and the newer Queen Elizabeth Hospital out in Edgbaston. Here we would work in various wards for a period of time, then have another two weeks of lectures and study, and meet again at the Children's Hospital for another month. Then we would spend the remainder of the three years at the two major hospitals, the Nerve Hospital and the Women's Hospital, with 'study blocks' of a couple of weeks in between.

During that time we would have many exams; finishing with major Hospital and National ones. Throughout, our constant companion was a little cardboard covered booklet issued by the General Nursing Council for England and Wales, which was a comprehensive record of practical instruction and experience. Inside, columns of all the techniques we were expected to perform were listed, with the signature of the relevant Ward Sister as indication of our proficiency. Subjects were as varied as ward management, general patient care, bed making, giving and removing bedpans and urinals, giving injections, collecting measuring and charting body fluids, giving and receiving reports on patients, administration of drugs, giving injections, administration of oxygen, surgical techniques, bandaging, positions needed for nursing care, recording and reporting on patients' condition, catheterisation, removal of sutures, pre and post operative care, operating theatre experience, and sterilising and laying many trolleys for surgical procedures, to name just a few.

I was only to be on the women's medical ward for two weeks and it was a gentle introduction. The Sister was a beautiful woman, with a figure which even the austere navy-blue uniform could not hide. I noted frequent visits by several of the younger doctors in the time I was there. I suppose I had a bit of a crush on her and wished one day I would be like her.

She was gentle in her instruction and not overly critical of the classical mistakes I made. One, which later I delighted in seeing in the film *'Carry on Nurse'*, involved a contraption for cleaning bedpans. It was fixed on the wall, with a hinged lid, into which the soiled pan was slotted. The nurse then closed the lid and locked it firmly in place. A handle at the side was then pulled hard to send a strong jet of water to wash out the pan. If the lock was not properly in place the jet flung the lid open again, drenching the poor unsuspecting nurse. It was a common sight to see the newest nurses walking dripping out of the sluice room, much to the amusement of the patients. As in the film, I almost lost my spectacles down the drain.

The other classical mistake again involved bedpans. In those days the only way to sterilise them was to boil them in a huge sterilizer. After being cleaned, they were then stacked in this tank-like contraption, and it was filled with water from a tap. This took ages, and usually there were so many things to do, a nurse did not have time to stand and wait. It was quite a regular occurrence to see the tide of water slowly seeping out from under the sterilising room door, and a red-faced junior nurse hurrying to turn off the forgotten tap.

I must have made an impression with my first ward sister, as she gave me a small, enamelled brooch like a rose, which I still have in my jewellery box.

After a couple of weeks I was moved to a male surgical ward. We junior nurses soon learned to look at the nurses' home notice board as movement from one ward to another was quite frequent, to allow us as much varied experience as possible. This new ward was a baptism of fire for me. I had been lulled into a false sense of security, tending to the needs of mostly elderly long-term women patients. The men in my new ward were there for shorter terms; hernia repairs, varicose vein stripping and some more serious cases with gastric, prostate and liver surgeries. The first patient I had to deal with, literally as I walked into the ward, caused my innocent eighteen-year-old face to burn with embarrassment.

'Nursey, Nursey, can you come and help?' The face peeping round the drawn bedside curtain was of a young attractive red-headed man. I looked up the ward, but no other nurse was in sight, so I slipped in behind the curtain. He was sitting on the edge of the bed, wearing just a pyjama top. I realised the dressing was from a circumcision. As I backed out I nearly collided with a dressing trolley wheeled by the Staff Nurse. 'Ah, you're the new first year. Atkinson, isn't it? Well, you can do this.' I felt sorry for the poor young man, as I was not very proficient or I fear gentle, but I had to learn.

The several weeks I was on that ward gave me more than physical experience. I had not had many dealings with the opposite sex, except my brother's friends, but I found my uniform gave me a sort of glamour. These patients were generally full of fun, and soon they latched on to the brisk walk I cultivated to cover my lack of experience. Some wit would start to whistle the theme tune from the Laurel and Hardy films, and the rest would follow suit. I learned to tease the younger men and chatted with the older ones who often reminded me of my father. I also enjoyed learning to do the dressings and was given instruction by the Staff Nurse. It had always been my job to patch up my brother or our cats and dog, if they were hurt, so I was used to it.

All too soon my time was ended on this ward, but not entirely, as next we were moved to night duty. The hours were long, from 9.30pm to 8am, and lasted for several months at a time. I had become used to the daytime shifts, and if there was a sympathetic Sister, you would have a duty from 8am to 4pm before your one day off a week, and not start again until 4pm the day after. The worst shift was a split one. On duty at 8am; off at 12, then back again at 3pm and off again at 9pm. It was impossible to do anything else with the day.

It was always a dilemma when starting night duty, whether to try and sleep during the day before starting that evening when you had slept the night before, or to stick it out. Eventually you became used to the strange half-life, emerging at the end like an animal from hibernation.

Meals were odd, too. There was no provision for our topsy turvy time scale, so we had to become used to dinner as we went on duty, instead of breakfast, and a fry-up instead of dinner.

I was first pleased to have a while on the male surgical ward I had just finished as a daytime nurse, but I was soon moved on. Night nurses had to be prepared to move around, and in my three months, I worked on the women's and a men's orthopaedic wards, women's surgical, venereal diseases ward, with private patients, and finally on casualty and the adjoining casualty ward.

This last was quite a different experience, and my first night was one I was to remember for some time.

3

By the time I was moved to Casualty, I thought I had gained enough experience not to be fazed by whatever presented itself.

I was to learn differently.

'Nurse, go along to cubicle two will you. There's an old man there needs to have a history taken. He's been in before; likes his drink a bit too much.'

I smelled the beer before I even pulled the curtain aside to step in. It was mixed with unwashed body odour and I could see the old man was a vagrant. A soiled bag was pushed in the corner, containing his worldly possessions. He was still dressed in a shabby old coat tied with string round the waist, and his hair was straggly and matted and he badly needed a shave. I felt sorry for him and wondered how he had ended like this on the street. Whose son was he? Did he have a family or friends?

Walking over I saw he had his eyes closed and wondered how I was going to take details from him, when he suddenly sat up. His eyes opened and he stared at me, unseeing for a moment, then a jet of vomit narrowly missed me and he slumped back onto the stretcher bed with a groan. Stepping round the unpleasant puddle on the floor, I realised he was unconscious and tried to turn him over so he would not choke, but looking at his pallid face and staring eyes I realised it was too late: the old man was already dead. Just to be sure I searched for a pulse, feeling so sad that a life should have ended in this way.

The Staff Nurse in charge was sympathetic, but also very busy. 'Have you done Last Offices yet nurse?' At my nod, she looked undecided. 'You should really have someone with you, but I just don't have a spare nurse. Can you cope?' I swallowed hard and nodded again.

I had laid out the dead several times before, and as I was a Christian and believed there was something else beyond, I knew I would be able to manage. It was not the pleasantest job to perform, but somehow it was done, but I was glad of the strong cup of coffee the Staff Nurse offered me at a short break.

Nursing in Casualty was very different from any other of my experiences. Often it was full on and sometimes there were literally life and death situations. In between emergencies work was freer, with little barrier between the seniority of the nurses and doctors. This was because we all had to pull our weight in the situations in which we nightly found ourselves. I greatly enjoyed my time there and gained in confidence, becoming friendly with a few student doctors, as the hospital group was used for doctor's training in conjunction with the Birmingham University, situated close to the Queen Elizabeth Hospital.

It was also my introduction to student parties, being sucked into the social life by Patsy. We had stayed friends despite our different natures, although I had discovered a wilder side to my own personality, previously hidden by my strict upbringing. My fair hair had grown longer as it was easier to manage under the starched cap, and I had discovered makeup when off duty, which was not allowed when wearing uniform.

It was at one of these parties I made friends with a group of dental students who were housed in the Dental Hostel opposite the General Hospital. They were a mad lot, and on more than one occasion when I was back on day duty, I would whizz through the city in a sports car owned by one, after an all-night party, to change into uniform and report straight for morning duty. Thankfully I was never caught.

I was to be grateful to these students for years to come as I volunteered to be a 'patient' for dental treatment, especially in their exams. The work would have to be perfect, and I acquired several gold inlays which lasted for many years. The disadvantage, when they were practicing with my mouth wide open for long periods, was my inability to answer their teasing. We had fun times, but I never became emotionally involved with any of them. These were the days before 'the pill' and even if tempted, the fear of pregnancy made sure I was one of the 'good girls.' Anyway I had met Ken who was to be my future husband.

At the end of night duty we were awarded the luxury of two weeks' holiday to be followed by a 'study block' then a spell in the children's hospital. I decided I would treat myself to a pony trekking holiday run by the Youth Hostel Association. I had been a member for a few years, receiving issues of a small magazine. In one of these I saw the advertisement for a pony trekking holiday of a week centring in Tavistock in Dartmoor and to ride over the moor for a night in a remote Youth Hostel. It sounded something I would really enjoy. I had been horsed-mad since I could remember, but never owned a horse or pony, but had worked in a stable near my grammar school in a village called Shottery. I had first spent my pocket money on lessons, but then offered to work there for no wages. I learned the hard way, as it was my duty to ride the kinks out of the frisky ponies before the children of the wealthy arrived for their lessons.

I had also persuaded an elderly woman in the village where I lived, to let me ride her pet pony. I had seen it day after day in the field opposite my parents' cottage, never being ridden. One day I took courage and walked up the drive of the large house and knocked on the door.

'Good morning Mrs Winter, I live over the road in 'Four Winds;' I was wondering if you would like your pony exercised.' Here my courage failed me a little especially as her nasty little Corgi was nipping at my heel. At <u>first</u> I paid to ride, but then I saw a lovely little governess cart in her shed, and I offered to paint it, as it was a little shabby, and then I had free rides.

Eventually she taught me how to drive and harness the pony, which later was to be very useful.

There were eight of us on the pony trekking holiday: two men and 6 girls and surprisingly both men were called Ken: Ken G and Ken D. Both admitted they had not ridden before, and I thought them very brave, if a little foolhardy. The other girls were mostly like myself; keen riders but without their own horse or pony, and we were led by a young man who irritated me at first by making a smart comment at my expense. On the application form we had to say what experience we had, and this cocky fellow remarked I must be a bit sore by now as I had written *'I have been riding since I was 13.'* I forgave him later as the pony he selected for me was a darling, though a bit feisty.

Having gained experience with my dentist friends, I had become comfortable with male company and enjoyed both Kens. The younger, Ken G was quite intense and latched on to me, but it was the other, and darkly handsome one I really fancied. He had wonderful wavy hair and eyelashes to die for, but seemed a little shy. Determined to bring him out of his shell I spent time teasing him and goading him to respond. After a while, he did relax more, and on one occasion when I had been particularly obnoxious, locked me in the broom cupboard; sadly not with him.

It was a wonderful holiday. The terrain we rode over was mainly moorland and it was exhilarating to gallop over the heather strewn hills with the wind in our hair, although I always felt a little less in control with the faster pace. Poor Ken D had been given a large heavier mount called Satan, who did not live up to his name, with no fire in his soul. He was always a hill behind with Ken urging him on with little effect, yelling *'Come on Satan,'* to our great amusement.

At the end of the holiday Ken G asked to keep in touch, although he lived in London, many miles from Birmingham. Ken D also lived in London, and I was determined to keep in touch with him too. We all exchanged addresses and phone numbers, and I returned to the hospital world planning how to visit London as soon as I could.

4

The study block prior to our next few weeks duty, was focused on children's illnesses before we were let loose in the Children's Hospital. I was not looking forward to this as I hated to think of little ones being ill enough to be in hospital. We then had to move temporarily to a nurses' home in an area called Ladywood and I was pleased to have a small room to myself

I was not so happy to be sent first to a chronic illness ward. Some were 'hole in the heart' babies waiting for operations to rectify their birth defects. I remembered a lecture we had just been given on that very subject.

'Before birth a foetus has certain peculiarities in the heart and lungs, bypassing the need for the lungs to be operative in the womb,' we were told. 'These should always disappear with the first breath of the new-born, thus allowing the lungs and heart to function normally.'

A student asked, 'Is that why it is so important to make the baby cry as soon as it is born?'

The lecturer continued. 'Yes indeed, and it has sometimes been a way to determine if a baby a mother claimed was stillborn, was in fact alive when born.'

'Who would do that?'

'The pressure of too many children in poorer areas has sometimes been a factor.'

We silently looked at each other with sadness. As young women hoping to have children one day, the thought was sobering.

'One of these abnormalities,' he added, is called a *'Ventricular Septum Defect'* when the wall between the lower left and right sides in the heart, the ventricles, maintained a small hole, which should have closed. This means the rich blood full of oxygen from the lungs which should be pumped to the organs of the body, becomes contaminated with deoxygenated blood.'

I was to see several of these little children in the next few weeks. They were usually pale and underweight, with lacklustre eyes and thin cries. Sometimes we had to help the doctor taking blood samples from veins in the scalp which must have been very painful, poor mites. At other times I had to take them for a procedure called *'cardiac catheterisation,'* when a very fine radio-opaque catheter was inserted into one of the child's veins to pass through the heart and be x-rayed. I was very happy to be moved on to the baby ward.

These little babies were not so ill; mostly in for medical circumcisions, hernia operations and similar surgery. Much of my time was spent in making up feeds and giving them to the infants.

The Staff Nurse, Janet, was one I had worked with in my first weeks in the Women's Medical ward as a 'Final Year Nurse.' She had passed her exams and opted to stay on for a fourth year as a junior Staff Nurse. This was compulsory if you wanted to be awarded your 'Queen Elizabeth School of Nursing Badge'; a much coveted red, silver and black oval, with the motto *'Health, Teach, Learn,'* and a stylised crown and figures embossed on it. We had become friends as she had been to the 'Hugh Clopton Grammar School' in Stratford-on-Avon before me, and we had memories in common, so we spent some time chatting when not busy.

'Chris,' she said one morning break, as we had a cup of tea. 'You will be in your second year very soon. Have you thought of living out? Because if you have, would you like to share with me? My other flat mate is getting married.'

Of course, I had been looking forward to living in a flat or bedsit as soon as I could, but did I want to share again? As accommodation was expensive in Birmingham, with the nurses and university students as well looking for a place to live, I decided to see what was on offer.

Janet knew I was not keen to share but said she would soon be on night duty for a few weeks, and as I was on 'days' we would not see much of each other so I made a date to view the flat with her the next time we had time off together.

It was right at the top of a rambling old house in the suburb of Edgbaston, with a bus stop outside, so getting to work would not be too difficult. We climbed up a steep flight of steps and I wondered if we were going up onto the roof, but finally Janet pulled out her key, warning me to step back as the door opener outwards. The room was small and a large double bed took up a good part, but the view over the rooftops was dramatic through the windows which took up most of one wall.

'There is even a small kitchen, and we share a bathroom with just one other tenant.' Janet showed me a cubicle with small basin, a meat safe and two gas rings. It was not luxury, but the rent was reasonable, and I decided on the spot it would do for a start. At least I would be independent and could come and go as I pleased.

I had contacted Ken G as promised and he seemed keen for me to visit him in London but I delayed until the move out of the Nurses' Home. I had also written to Ken D, and he had replied, indicting if I was ever in London, to look him up.

For a while my time was taken with study for the end of the first year exams. These were two-fold, as were all our exams; both State and Hospital. I studied hard as I certainly did not wish to be sent home after just one year. While my decision to become a nurse was almost by default, there being little other alternative, by this time I knew it was what I wanted to do more than anything else. I found people fascinating, and in the hospital environment most were reduced to their true selves; pretensions discarded while needing help and reassurance. I had also become interested in the different attitudes people had to illness. Those with a positive outlook seemed to progress more favourably than the 'cup half empty' types. So often I had noticed two patients with similar diagnosis and prognosis on a ward would respond so differently to the treatment. The relaxed, friendly and extrovert type seemed to recover so much more quickly than the other who was always worried, depressed and anxious.

I passed my exams reasonably well, and at last was able to fix the blue epaulets on my buttercup yellow uniform to denote my status as a second-year student nurse. As soon as I could I moved out to my little shared attic bedsit, and made plans to visit London, and the two Kens.

At the end of our time in the Children's Hospital our PTS, which had been split originally between the General Hospital in the city centre and the Queen Elizabeth Hospital in Edgbaston, were now changed over. I was delighted to begin my second year in a much more modern hospital. First we were all given a weekend off and I wasted no time in booking into a Youth Hostel in the centre of London.

Ken G met me at the railway station and was as intense as I remembered him on holiday, keenly giving me my first view of the city's tourist spots. He tried to hold my hand, which I was not too keen on as it was hot and sweaty. Then when we found ourselves alone in a part of Hampstead Heath he grabbed and kissed me. As we both wore glasses they clinked together and made me giggle which I think annoyed him as he became more persistent, pressing his body onto mine. By this time I was not totally ignorant about the opposite sex and realised Ken G was fired up and passionate wanting more than just the friendship I thought we had.

'You shouldn't have led me on, Chris. I thought you wanted a relationship, as you came all this way to see me.'

I had not the heart to say it was really Ken D I wanted to meet up with and returned guiltily to the Youth Hostel. Having learned my lesson I returned to Birmingham without contacting Ken D and threw myself into the beginning of my second year. I had been put on Theatre duty.

5

The modern Queen Elizabeth Hospital boasted up to date equipment especially in the theatres. Some of the more complicated procedures were performed there and I was a little nervous about becoming a theatre nurse. My first day arrived, and I presented myself at the allotted time to be met by a thin Staff Nurse who made it clear she had little time for inexperienced juniors. I knew she had been on the theatre staff there for many years, always trying to ascend to the position of a Charge Sister, but never quite making it. This had turned her sour and she usually took it out of the newest nurses. I knew I was in for a hard time but decided to try and ignore her attitude. I had also been told by other students, if I showed an aptitude, she could be very helpful. For now she just snapped;

'Hurry up and change into your greens nurse in that locker room. Then come into theatre...and don't forget the overshoes and a mask. There's a below knee amputation on at the moment and the surgeon Sir Thomas Spraggs doesn't like noise, so keep out of the way.'

With that she slipped through the theatre doors and left. Fortunately when I had been on Casualty there had been a small theatre attached where my assistance was needed. I was familiar with the green cotton square necked dresses, elasticised caps and overshoes, so managed to change quickly. I had discovered a way to stop my glasses steaming up while I was wearing a mask in Casualty as well, so I quickly rubbed soft soap on the lenses and wiped it off, leaving a thin film.

Finally I was ready, and with heart beating, slid into the theatre. I could hear the bone saw humming and felt a little sick while I quietly approached the activity. I had seen the surgeon during his ward rounds, and then had thought him a little like the actor James Roberson Justice in his outspoken and loud manner. Now he looked up quickly as I moved, then flicked his eyes to the nurse by his side, to have his brow wiped.

The leg had now been separated from the patient, and lay there on the operating table, while the doctor and his assistant tied blood vessels and built a flap over the raw area. Looking up again, Sir Thomas caught my eye and shouted, 'Well get rid of the bloody leg, nurse. This isn't a side show.'

Still feeling a little sick, I stepped forward and grabbed the offending article, wrapped in the green operating towels, and stood there for a moment not knowing what to do with it. Everyone else was intent on the activity round the table and offered no help until a nurse whispered; 'down the chute.' Glancing over to one side I saw the sterilising room and two stainless steel chutes so made my way there. Wanting to get rid of my burden as soon as possible I shot it, towels and all down the nearest one. Only then did I see one had *'City Dump'* and the other *'Incinerator'* written on them. I had sent the dismembered leg to the city dump and had a fleeting vision of police looking for the rest of the body.

This was a gruesome introduction but I was not generally squeamish, having been given the job as a child to clear up after pet cats and dogs, but this was a little different. The theatre was a busy one, dealing often with major surgery and soon I was involved in sterilising and laying up the instrument trolleys. Most of the instruments had to be boiled or sterilised in an autoclave, and we nurses had to learn which order each surgeon liked them displayed.

Usually the 'main scrub' .... the senior Sister or Staff Nurse assisting ... needed to know the peculiarities of each surgeon. We had to learn the different glove sizes of each surgeon too and present them on a sterile towel for him to put on. It was quite an exercise as a surgeon arrived in the 'scrub room' prior to commencing his work. He would already have on his mask, clinical cap and white waterproof boots. First he would wash and clean his hands and forearms with the provided equipment, drying them on sterilised towels. A nurse would hand him a sterile gown by forceps and he would don this, careful not to contaminate it. Another nurse would tie the ribbons at the back without contaminating him, and finally on went the gloves.

The first assistant nurse would be gowned similarly and there were other 'scrubs' as they were called, to assist in threading needles etc. Later on I was promoted to this job, which was quite onerous. It was difficult to hold the needle, often curved, in a pair of forceps and with gloved hand, thread catgut or silk sutures into the small hole, and then hand it all to the waiting Sister who would be standing impatiently watching. Catgut was mostly used internally as it eventually dissolved, and the silk for skin closures. As my hands were small, I seldom had a pair of gloves to fit properly, often leaving me with a small bubble at the end of each finger which hindered efficiency.

For the first few weeks, as the most junior, I had the most menial jobs; mopping blood from the floors and picking up anything else a surgeon decided to throw down, and cleaning and sterilising stainless steel bowls and instruments. Gradually I was trusted to prepare the 'runabouts' needed in all operations. These were two stainless steel bowls in a carrier on wheels, one inverted onto the other, with receivers and gallipots inside. It was a tricky job removing the boiling hot bowl from the large steriliser with a special type of 'Cheatle forceps'; setting it carefully in the runabout on wheels, then placing the receivers inside and finally lifting the second bowl and inverting it onto the first to keep all sterile inside. I had to practice this privately when there were no operations taking place and became quite adept.

Until one day just before Sir Thomas was due to start his list.

I had just performed the ritual and had turned round to close the steriliser lid when there was an almighty crash behind be. I could not believe I had made a mistake, and spun round, only to see the surgeon standing with his hands on his hips, glaring at me.

'There, nurse. If you did that when I was operating, I could cut a bloody artery!'

I was incensed and spoke without thinking. 'I don't do it when you are operating and now I've got to sterilise the bloody lot again.'

There was a deadly silence, and then it was split by a mighty guffaw; Sir Thomas Spraggs had a sense of humour. I knew I would be summoned to Sister's office, but fortunately the surgeon had taken a fancy to me and had said a word in my favour. The next day when I reported for duty the Staff Nurse was waiting for me and almost smiled in approval, 'Quick, Atkinson. Get prepared to assist. The student doctors are in exams and Sir Thomas has asked for you.'

I felt very nervous as I had discovered I did not have a very good tolerance of the sight of blood and I would be right there where it was all happening. In reality, for all his gruffness, the surgeon was a good teacher and his instructions took my mind off my problem. I never became quite accustomed to the first swipe of the razor-sharp scalpel as the skin separated like a sudden opening mouth, with the granular bubble of sub coetaneous fat underneath, but it was my job to hold the wound open with retractors...sort of big clamps... so I had no time to think about it. Having secured these then the blood which welled into the cavity had to be removed, either with a suction device or using large gauze 'swabs.' Each time one of these was used, a nurse had to put a tally up on a blackboard. At the end of the operation, before the wound was sutured closed, all these swabs needed to be accounted for. The danger was to have one left in the wound.

It was also my job to clamp any small blood vessel if told to. I became used to the direction; 'Clamp the bleeder, nurse.' and became fascinated to see the inside of the patient. I was given considerable instructions on the various organs and so was very sorry when the trainee doctors returned and I had to revert to more menial chores. As I left theatre after my final shift there, I was pleased to overhear Sir Thomas Spraggs shouting to one student. 'That young nurse is more use than you, young man. Clamp the bloody bleeder.'

6

My next move was to a ward with private paying patients and it caused me a little anxiety. Stories had been circulated of how difficult some patients could be and to crown this I was to have another stint there on night duty. My flat-mate Janet was going on holiday for two weeks then back on day duty, so at least we would not have to share the double bed. It took a little while to get used to Janet arriving tired from her spell on night duty, ready for the bed I had just vacated.

So far the flat had worked well, but I realised I would need to look for somewhere else soon as the tiny room and lack of proper cooking facilities became a handicap. The absence of a fridge was a particular disadvantage, as was soon apparent.

The private ward was a series of individual rooms, eh with the luxury of an en-suite bathroom. We nurses had an office and there was a small well equipped and supplied kitchen which surprised me, and I asked the day sister about it when reporting for duty.

'You will find these patients expect special treatment, Nurse Atkinson. If they can't sleep they will expect a snack prepared for them and we can't call on the main kitchen too often. Can you cook?' Nodding, I blessed my mother for training me from an early age.

Some of the patients were quite ill but several had minor ailments like in-growing toenails or bunion removal. These were the most demanding; expecting sandwiches, an omelette or even bacon and eggs at all hours of the night, despite having consumed a luxurious evening meal. Occasionally something was left over from the supper, and rather than throw away good food it found its way to our various flats. Such was a tasty piece of ham one night, so we split it to take home. Not fancying it when I went off duty it was put it in the meat safe, where it lay forgotten for a couple of days. I had been feeling a little unwell with the start of a cold and decided to make myself a tasty sandwich before going on duty. I opened the safe's door to see the pink meat crawling with maggots. A bluebottle must have discovered it. By the time I had cleared the mess I realised I would be late to go on duty that night, and the bed looked very inviting. I had not had any time off sick, so had no guilt in walking down to the hall and phoning the Night Sister. In my best Birmingham accent said 'I'm phoning fur Miss Atkinson; she's not well, y'know and can't come in t'night.'

That decided me, and I started to look for a place with more facilities.

It was a custom that anyone offering accommodation would advertise on the Nurses Home notice board. For some time I had been popping in to the Home to see what was on offer, but usually anything worthwhile was snapped up quickly as residents had first pickings. So the decision was made to look elsewhere.

On the next appointment with my dental student pals, when I could close my mouth enough to talk, I mentioned my search. 'If you don't mind sharing a kitchen with us, we do have a spare bedroom, Chrissie...' I must have looked a little sceptical; 'No hanky panky, I promise; we all have girlfriends, or, er boyfriends, if you're OK with that?'

I had become used to the sexual preferences of some of the young students by this time, although I was a little uncomfortable with it, but my philosophy was 'live and let live.'

I moved into the large Victorian house in Edgbaston as soon as possible, and it was such an improvement. My room was high ceilinged and airy, looking out onto the overgrown garden. It was Spring again, with daffodils showing in the long grasses of a neglected lawn and delightful with the bright green of young oak leaves.

Sparse furniture was supplied in my room; a single bed, an old wooden wardrobe, a chair and a mirror on the wall, but it was home. On visits to my parents I eventually acquired a few comforts; a sheepskin rug, better curtains, some cushions and a few pictures. One or two were my own sketches, as I had continued with my love of drawing, when I had time.

There was a large communal kitchen, a sitting room, and two bathrooms. As I was on night duty for the first few weeks, I had the place almost to myself, although it took me a while to accustom myself to the chatter and banging doors while I was trying to sleep during the day when others were off duty. Getting used to the 'kitchen roster' was another new experience. There were two other women, sharing occasionally with their boyfriends, but they did not help much in keeping the kitchen tidy. We were supposed to take it in turns, but men being men, sometimes they needed a reminder to clear up after themselves.

We each put our names on our personal food in the fridge, and woe betide anyone who 'stole' another's goodies. Occasionally we had a communal meal, each contributing and it was a revelation to me to socialise so much with other young people. It did much to give me confidence in mixing, but I was always a bit of a loner making no really close friends, except Patsy.

We had kept in touch occasionally when we changed wards and had both moved to the Queen Elizabeth Hospital at the same time. One morning as I sat over my meal of bacon, eggs and fried bread, thinking it would be a relief to get back to proper meals at the right time, she plonked herself on the seat opposite.

'When are you off nights, Chris?'

'A couple of weeks; why?'

'Let's go to the student's hop at the university. D'you dance?'

I nodded; remembering my two month's stay with relatives in Bridlington before I became old enough to start my training. There was a huge Spa ballroom, complete with revolving mirrored sphere, where I had learned to waltz, quickstep and jive; and had loved it. I remembered fondly the ritual when we girls arrived. We would sit or stand to one side of the large room and the boys were on the other side, eyeing each other. I always worried I would be a 'wallflower' but after I had been invited once or twice, my ability to follow my partner in the dance moves, made me almost popular. I was looking forward to another chance to show off my expertise.

'How do we get in, I thought you had to be escorted by a student?'

Patsy just grinned at me. 'Ways and means; ways and means, Chris. We'll make a date.'

Coming off night duty, nurses were usually given a day to recover and then not be on duty until the four pm shift the next day. My change was over the weekend, so Patsy and I made a plan to go dancing.

Dressed in our best, we made our way to the main door of the Student's Union building. I had been as usual dissatisfied with my lack of a bosom, so had bought a padded bra and felt particularly fetching, as I had abandoned my spectacles as well. I figured I did not need sharp eyesight to dance.

As we approached, Patsy pulled me to one side; 'The plan is, you wait until you see a man on his own or with a friend and you persuade them to take you in. If you don't like them, you can easily give them the slip once you are inside.'

It wasn't long before we saw two students approaching, and so we stepped forward, asking if they would escort us. 'And where do you come from, girls?'

'We're nurses,' I blurted out and winced as Patsy pinched me and I realised I had said the wrong thing. When we were inside we made an excuse to visit the Ladies' toilet.

Patsy frowned at me; 'Chris, you are a twit. They all think nurses are fair game. You get the "bedroom" look as soon as they realise. Come on we'd better lose them.'

It did not prove too easy for me, but Patsy was an old hand and somehow managed to go off on her own. I was stuck with a pimply young man with terrible breath who offered to get me a drink. After the glass of wine, I felt it would be rude to refuse at least one dance so accepted. It was a quickstep, and my partner had some idea what to do, but held me far too close. It was as we parted a little during a corner, I heard a distinct "pop" as one of my padded bra cups righted itself after being crushed. I could not help myself and started to giggle, especially when I saw my partner's startled expression.

'I'm sorry....I have to go...' and dashed to the Ladies' again. After a while I re-joined the dancers and enjoyed the evening and fortunately did not see my previous partner again. I hoped I had not caused him too much alarm.

I had not seen Patsy since we separated, but eventually I decided to walk back to my flat. It was a clear night, and after the smoky dance hall it was refreshing. Walking through the quiet streets I felt very alone and a little lonely, and this was made more acute by the occasional un-curtained window, with the lights showing life revealed in little cameos. I was a stranger looking in to lives of which I had no part and made me wonder what lay ahead for me.

7

My time on the private ward was short as we were due once more for two weeks of study block before working in the Women's' Hospital for a spell. We were to have a few days holiday between the study block and our duty, so I decided to visit London again. I had taken the courage to write to Ken D and we had been exchanging letters for some time. He told me he worked for a large company in their advertising department, having studied in night school to become a junior manager. Due to the bombing of London in the Second World War he had had to leave school at age of fifteen with few qualifications but had been determined to better himself. He told me also he was very keen on classical music, writing a music report frequently in a column in a North London paper. This floored me a little as the only classical music in my family had been two records with parts of *'Eine Kleine Nachtmusik'* and *'Fingal's Cave,'* but I was willing to learn.

I booked to stay at the same Youth Hostel in London and was a little nervous about meeting Ken D again. The holiday was a while ago, and I wondered if I had been glamourising Ken in the interim, but when I saw him again, my heart flipped a little. His dark wavy hair and eyes gave a foreign look and he seemed so much more mature than the young men I had befriended. True, he was rather serious and seldom smiled, but I suspected he was as nervous as I was. He took me around the London sights and was a perfect gentleman, making no passes at me and only giving me a chaste kiss on the lips, which if I were honest was less than I had hoped for. He was a man of twenty-eight, and I was still only just nineteen, but I thought myself falling in love. We made plans to meet again when I had a weekend off.

'I'd like you to come and meet my parents Chris. Would you come and stay in the spare room, do you think?'

I was a little surprised: things were moving too fast, but I agreed.

The lectures in the study block had been mainly on gynaecology, with a little on obstetrics, but not midwifery. The patients were mostly in hospital after various operations; tubal ligation; hysterectomy; complications of childbirth, and sadly several with cancer, often of the breast. I remembered for the rest of my life, one thing a lecturer said. Sweeping his gaze around the eighty or so students, he declared;

'I would expect at least fifty percent of you will have cancer of one sort or another in your lifetime, particularly of the breast. It is imperative you learn how to self-examine regularly'

After my short break in London it was straight on duty in the Women's Hospital and my life was busy. Many of the patients were not in very long, as operations like tubal ligation...tying of the fallopian tubes to prevent pregnancy...did not require long hospitalisation. This meant bed linen changes and thorough cleaning of the beds and lockers was frequent, as was organising the discharge of one patient and the admission of another. We junior nurses were responsible for all this, as well as post operative care.

One of the frequent complications of minor abdominal operations was the interference with normal body functions, and patients must have passed urine and had a bowel movement before they were cleared for discharge, to make sure everything was working normally. As I sometimes had a similar problem, with a changed and somewhat irregular diet, on research I had discovered swinging back and forward while trying to function, increased the *peristalsis*...the natural movement of the intestines.

The ladies normally were given a bedpan which they placed on a bedside chair or the side of the bed for comfort. One day I mentioned my idea to a young woman who was having a little difficulty, and thought no more of it for a while.

A day or so after this conversation, as I entered the ward I heard gales of laughter and the unmistakable the strains of *'Swing low sweet chariot,'* wafting to greet me. I peeped into see the patient I had told my idea, and she laughingly said she had passed it on. I am not sure if it worked, but at least it had caused some merriment.

Amusement was certainly needed in some cases. Young women with breast cancer were frequent patients and some happily appeared to be controlled...we were told not to think of the word 'cured'...while sometimes they returned with metastases, or 'secondary carcinoma.' I was relieved when my time was over at this hospital, feeling constantly 'there but for the grace of God, go I.' It was very difficult emotionally to disassociate yourself from patients sometimes, especially when some were not much older than I was.

My next move was back to the General Hospital in the centre of Birmingham where I had started. This time I was on an orthopaedic ward, looking after patients who mostly had been in accidents with broken bones. Some of the contraptions looked like medieval torture devices and I felt sorry for the young men strung up in them. It was not my favourite ward, as nursing the bedridden patients was very hard work, and I never did get the hang of the various types of treatments and bed setup necessary. At the time I was grateful to spend only a few weeks there, before our final move to the Nerve Hospital but had reason to regret the lack of my knowledge of orthopaedics when eventually I took my final exams.

The previous study block covered various psychiatric disorders and I was not looking forward to that either. I was into night duty, which was, I thought, going to be easier, turned out to be anything but. For a start I was in sole charge of the male ward. Most of the patients were well sedated and all I had to do was the drug round with the day sister before she went off duty. Prior to that I had to take the hot drinks trolley round offering Horlicks and hot chocolate, but not coffee or tea, as they were regarded as too stimulating. Then there was a bedpan and urinal round for the few patients who could not get up. Finally I walked round the sleeping patients, checked the outside door to the conservatory was locked, as the ward was on the ground floor.

The rest of the night was spent in rolling cotton wool balls and folding gauze squares for sterilisation in the hospital's autoclave; this was traditionally the night nurses' job.

I did find I was able to catch up on my study, as we were soon to take major exams at the end of our second year. Occasionally a patient would wake up and complain he could not sleep and ask for another pill. I had been warned about this by the night Sister.

'Everyone has the correct medication, so what we find works is a nice milky drink and you can give them an ascorbic acid...vitamin C tablet...from the drugs cupboard. Tell them it is a mild sleeping pill.' I thought this was a little like cheating, but I did find it worked when accompanied by a sympathetic ear. All went well for the first week and I began to feel a little more confident.

Then we had the visit from the Police.

There were two constables in uniform talking to the day staff nurse as I reported for duty at the beginning of my second week.

'Ah, nurse Atkinson, just in time.' The staff nurse gave a smile to the young policemen, who I had to admit were a pleasant change from the patients, and informed me they had come to warn us a man had escaped from the secure unit of a nearby prison.

'He is dangerous, nurse, so make sure your doors are locked and don't answer anyone trying to enter.' With a smile to the pretty Staff nurse and a nod to me, they left.

For once I had quite a busy night as I had to admit a couple of new patients, who were staying in overnight for observation, and forgot the policemen's visit. It was peaceful in the wee small hours when I was finally able to sit at the lit-up table in the middle of the ward. I felt a little like a captain of a ship on the floodlit bridge guiding my sleeping crew towards the morning.

Then I was aware of a light shining briefly through the windows, and remembered the visit by the policemen. I walked quietly down to the end of the ward, shading my own torchlight, entering the conservatory to check the door was properly locked. As I reached to the handle, there was a muffled snuffling on the other side and my heart gave a flip until I realised it was a police dog, and sat heavily on a nearby chair to recover. I stood up and saw the silhouette of a man standing in the door to the ward. I stood frozen for a moment, until the man spoke::it was one of the new patients.

'Nurse; I can't sleep...do you think you could give me something?'

8

The second-year exams were difficult, especially those set by the School of Nursing. The sister tutor explained; 'If you can pass the hospital exams, then the State ones will appear easier.' She also gave us a piece of advice which I was to remember when it came to the finals. 'A large part of your marks will hang on your practical exam. If you are asked a subject you are not comfortable with in the main questions, say so. You will lose a few marks but offer a subject you know well, and usually the examiner will test you on that.'

Before the exams I took another trip to London and accepted Ken D's invitation to stay at his parents' home in North Finchley. I was very nervous as I was not really sure of my feelings for Ken. To meet his parents was a big step and I was not comfortable with a possible deception that there was more in our relationship than existed.

It was a semi-detached house with a net curtained bay window and the traditional unused lounge kept for visitors, and the spare room at the front overlooking the quiet suburban street. They made me feel welcome and there was no suggestion there was anything expected, other than friendship between Ken and me. I had been a little surprised Ken, at 28 was still living at home with his parents, but as the house was large and he was an only child, I supposed it was a sensible arrangement. He was a hard worker, travelling into the city centre on the tube daily, and apparently often arriving home quite late. Elsie, his mother, patiently kept a hot meal for him, but I think he often ate out, and after that first weekend I understood why. Meals were something of an endurance as she had obviously been brought up in the tradition of boiling vegetables until they had a universal colour and consistency, and roasting the joint until it shrivelled to half the size.

I did find Elsie's strict Methodist outlook created a barrier I never quite penetrated. I think she was one of the few people I have met who had little if any sense of humour. The only time I knew her stiff restraint and quiet manner to relax was when Ken and I some years later gave her, by mistake, an alcoholic bottle of 'Stone's' ginger wine. We had been in the habit of giving the non-alcoholic version as a Christmas present and this particular Christmas was quite a jolly one.

Ken's builder father Bert and I became firm friends from that first visit. Small and tough, he had survived severe stomach ulcers and operations, which left him with little interest in the meals put in front of him; which I suppose was one of the reasons Elsie had no interest in cooking them.

'You see Chrissie...' I loved him to call me that... 'I only have a third of my stomach left.' He also told me he was not able to take painkillers like aspirin as it upset him. I had just discovered Paracetamol was kinder to the stomach and told him about it.

That first morning set a pattern which was to be for the next year. I first heard the whine of the milk cart and the clink as the two pint bottles were left on the doorstep. The door was opened quickly before the cheeky birds could peck through the foil lids and help themselves to the cream at the top. Then Elsie would quietly climb the stairs and deposit a strong cup of tea in the best rose-patterned china on my bedside table and wish me 'good morning.' I never had the heart to tell her I hated tea in bed!

After our second-year exams, we had a week's holiday, and after I spent a weekend with my parents I agreed to go on a cycling holiday with Ken, staying at Youth Hostels. I had bought myself a 'Moulton' bicycle and found the small wheels with the low centre of gravity made riding distances easy. This also left room on the carrier for my rucksack as well as some of Ken's gear. He had a 10-gear racing bike with less carrying space.

Being an outdoor girl, I revelled in travelling through the countryside, making our way across country and staying at some really unusual hostels. In those days there was no luxury; as there were separate dormitories for men and women in very basic bedrooms. Everyone was expected to accept some job or other set by the warden; helping prepare the communal meal, washing up after, or cleaning the rooms. If you did not do this then you had no meal. Everyone was also supposed to have a sheet sleeping bag, made of cotton with the pillowcase attached. You were lent a pillow and blankets. I never got the hang of it, as I usually woke with the pillow twisted on top of me and the sheet sleeping bag in a knot.

Many of the hostels were in unusual buildings. One was in an old wooden mill, and the men's dormitory was in what had been the grinding room, which was still covered in a fine film of flour. They all looked like ghosts as they staggered in for breakfast. Another was in St Briavels Castle in Gloucestershire where the dormitories were in the dungeons and there was no electricity; just candles.

After this holiday Ken and I became good friends, but I was still not sure if I wanted to become romantically attached to him: I had plans for my future, still wanting to travel and join the Queen Alexandra's Royal Army Nursing Corps with a commission after I qualified. We spent most of my time off together if I had a weekend free and inevitably romance grew from that friendship, but I was still rather young and had expected to be swept off my feet by Prince Charming. Ken was a restrained lover, never letting passion overcome his treatment of me. I had by this time learned a little about French kissing and 'heavy petting' and part of me wished my lover was less controlled, while I also realised he was being a perfect gentleman.

Gradually it was assumed we would marry, but I refused to be engaged until I had completed my three years' training, and Ken seemed content with this for the time being.

One interest Ken had was running a badminton youth club for youngsters from the less wealthy areas. It was housed in an old church hall which had been converted to a badminton court and small coffee bar. I had always been quite good at games so was happy to become involved and to learn how to play. The youngsters were mixed ages, from ten to seventeen and some were pretty rough. I became quite fond of several and we built a rapport which involved quite a lot of 'rough and tumble,' treating me like a big sister as I was more their age than Ken's.

The final year of training passed quickly, and I began to feel perfectly at home on whatever ward or department I was allocated. Sometimes I was asked to take a group of prospective 'would-be' nursing students around and marvelled at how young they all seemed, yet I was only twenty-one myself. I spent most of my time off with Ken. We had more youth hostel holidays, even hitch hiking on one. I would not have done this by myself of course, but it was safe with a man along. Then I took him up to meet my parents in Bridlington where they had moved after my father had been diagnosed with early Parkinson's' disease. That was a shock to me, but I had noticed he had not been his usual self for some time and complained of a weak right hand. There had been no tremor or I would have suspected it, but he did tend to stare into space and I later learned that was a peculiarity of the illness. He had also stopped writing the short stories he did so well, with moderate success. He had been put on medication and had improved, but decided to take early retirement and move up to his native Yorkshire.

I loved my father dearly; he was a gentle man, but ran his home on almost Victorian lines. His wife, Phyllis, our lovely step-mother, was expected to stay at home and care for the house and garden. My brother David and I had been brought up to respect him as head of the family, and we always were expected to accompany our parents on walks and cycle rides. To my brother this was a chore, as he was always studying, dragging behind with a book in his hands while I loved the outdoors.

The weekend with Ken was unremarkable, and he seemed to fit in with our middle-class lifestyle. It was only as we were leaving my father pulled me to one side.

'Chrissie, are you sure this is the man for you? '

9

For a while I was moved to work in the psychiatric ward in the Queen Elizabeth Hospital, which took the more acute cases. The equipment was more modern that that in the Nerve Hospital and included electroconvulsive therapy. While I had attended lectures about this procedure, which was calculated to help severe depression, maniac depression and schizophrenia by giving a brief electrical stimulation to the brain, I had never seen it used.

On my first day after the morning report the sister in charge asked me to stay behind.

'Nurse Atkinson, I want you to go with Maisie Brown for her treatment; have you done it before?' At my admission I had not, she said it would be good experience. 'The patient has a general anaesthetic, so you will need to attend to her before and after.'

I was still unprepared for what can only be described as a barbaric practice, akin to medieval torture. The patient was anaesthetised in a small room, not the theatre, with a rubber wedge placed between her teeth. When I asked why that was necessary, I was told;

'To stop the patient biting her tongue in half.'

What followed remained in my memory for years to come. An oblong box with electrical connections, a small window and various knobs was placed next to the unconscious patient. From this, two cables ran, with pads at the end. The doctor fiddled with the knobs, picked up the two cables and called 'charging; hold the patient,' while two student doctors held the patient's shoulders and legs. Quickly the doctor placed the pads either side of the patient's temples and pressed a switch on the machine. Immediately Maisie Brown convulsed violently, while the students constrained her and I looked on not knowing what I should be doing. This was soon made clear, as a breathing tube was substituted for the wedge and the patient was turned onto the recovery position on her side.

With a 'Stay with her, nurse,' the doctor and students left, saying they would call in a little later.

In a few moments the poor young woman spat the tube out and opened her eyes, looking totally confused. I had remembered reading there was often nausea after ECT, so was standing by with a bowl, which was needed.

I stayed with Maisie Brown, trying to comfort her, as she was finding it difficult to collect her thoughts, continually asking where she was and what had happened. I only hoped she would have some benefit from the treatment, as surely there was not much evidence of it at the time.

My stay on this ward was brief. I could not avoid the thought again, 'there but for the Grace of God, go I' when I saw the mental state of some of the patients. I always prided myself with being reasonably in control of my emotions, just occasionally giving way to, I had to admit, a slightly mercurial temperament. Though I did not really subscribe to believing in 'Zodiac signs,' and never read horoscopes in the papers, as a 'Sagittarian' I had discovered certain apparent personal peculiarities to that 'sign.' I loved the idea of travel and the excitement that would involve; I knew I was sometimes impatient when someone could not see a situation which to me was clear and I did possess some intuition and empathy. Which was why, on that ward, I could see how easily a person could tip over the edge from reality.

Soon the hospital exams were due, which were set a few weeks before the State finals. By passing all the State exams a student would eventually be a 'State Registered Nurse,' and entitled to use the qualification SRN. A pass in the hospital exams was needed if you wanted to continue for a fourth year as a staff nurse but did not affect the validity of the State exams.

As the day drew near for the written hospital exam, I was beginning to feel unwell. It was a cold foggy winter and I had to travel on public transport, so must have picked up some infection. I sneezed my way through the first papers, but decided I had better go to sick bay and get some medication.

The sister took my temperature and shook her head.

'Sorry; no way can you carry on with the practical exam; you'll spread your 'flu; and in any case I think you'll find you are too ill. Just go back to bed with aspirins and lots of liquids.'

I had no choice as I felt too ill to do other than fill my hot water bottle and snuggle down into my warm bed, sniffing and crying in frustration. The State exams were several weeks away, and so I had enough time to recover, spending my sick leave studying.

Although the exams were extensive, we were supposed to carry on working on the wards, and as luck would have it, I was sent on night duty again; this time on the ear, nose and throat ward. The work was not arduous but some of the procedures were very complicated. The surgeon specialised in ear problems and sometimes acute situations could flare up overnight and one such occurred a few days before I was due to take my practical exam. The procedure was a tympanostomy...the surgical perforation of the eardrum to release tension and often infection and pus. The attendant nurse needed to know all the complicated instruments the surgeon would need, sterilise them and lay them up on the trolley in the order the surgeon would require them. I had studied this so was able to organise this procedure successfully, which I was to be grateful for soon.

I was given a couple of days off before my practical State exam, as I was on night duty, and decided I was not going to try and cram any more knowledge into my brain, so I took myself to see the film 'Seven Brides for Seven Brothers.' I felt if I did not know what I needed to by then, it was too late. It was a welcome diversion and for the rest of my life I was to have a special affection for the songs sung by Howard Keel, Jane Powell and the rest of the cast.

It was only as I entered the examination room, my confidence wavered a little. There was an example ward situation with a dummy in a bed and shelves of instruments, several stainless-steel empty trolleys, and the stern supervisor standing by with a clipboard in her hand.

'Right,' she looked down at the clipboard, 'Nurse Atkinson, I want you to go over and make up that bed as a fracture bed.'

My mind went blank; I had spent little time on the orthopaedic ward, and I just could not remember how to do that. I could feel my face going red, then mercifully I remembered the advice our sister tutor had given us. Taking courage, I stammered; 'I am sorry but I have done little orthopaedics.'

'Hmm,' She looked down at the clipboard and made a mark...bang went five points. 'So what ward are you on now, nurse?'

I told her.

'Lay me up a tympanostomy trolley then.' I could have kissed her, and managed faultlessly to do that, earning a begrudging praise.

Relaxed then, I sailed through the rest of the practical exam.

10

Waiting for the results of the State exam was a nerve wracking experience, especially as I had to make a decision if I would take the hospital exams which I had missed, in a few months' time.

I was called to see the senior Matron.

'Nurse Atkinson, you have had very good reports from your various wards, and especially on theatre.' The thin face of the matron relaxed into a small smile. 'I understand you made an impression on Sir Thomas Spraggs particularly!' She looked down at her desk, 'I am assuming you wish to stay on as a fourth-year staff nurse? Maybe in theatre... but you will have to take your hospital exam as you were regrettably unwell, which means an extra six months. We need nurses of your calibre. I think you have a fulfilling future in the profession.'

I left the office in confusion, but with a warm feeling in my heart. I loved being a nurse, and particularly had enjoyed the day I had spent with a district nurse. From that experience had grown a conviction that was the sort of nurse I wanted to be; in the community. I had by now abandoned my plan to joining the QARANC as a pipe dream. Part of it had been a decision after a long chat with my stepmother. 'Chrissie, do you really think you could take all that discipline and kowtowing to the authority?' She knew I was a free spirit and even the hospital rules had irked me a little, but I endured as I had known they were only for three years. She was right. I think I would have balked at the hierarchy and constant saluting.

I was due some few days' leave, deciding to decide on my return and made plans to visit London again. It was approaching Valentine's Day and I looked forward to spending it with Ken and discussing my future, but I was very tired from the intensive exams and three years of training. Did I really want another six months of moving around the wards before I took yet more exams?

The decision was made for me.

Ken was particularly attentive; buying flowers and a pretty card which surprised and delighted me as he was not particularly romantic. The evening was one when we helped with the youth club, and I was touched by several of the youths giving me home-made Valentine cards. We took the tube train back to Finchley and as we walked home to his parents' house, Ken suddenly stopped me as we walked across the park.

'It is decision time, Chris. I have been very patient waiting for you to finish your training, but I am not prepared to stretch it to another eighteen months. Either we get engaged...or it is off.'

I stopped, shocked. I had been expecting some discussion, but I could see by Ken's face reflected in the streetlamp, he was deadly serious. We walked on in silence and I excused myself when we arrived at the house, saying I was tired.

I spent a wakeful night, going over and over in my mind what I really wanted to do. Many of my friends were engaged or married and the prospect of having my own home and a devoted husband was very appealing. The thought of possibly another long term of working in the hospital daunted me, and I could see myself being drawn permanently into that world.

But I was determined to train as a district nurse.

By morning I had decided, and at breakfast just said to Ken 'OK then, providing I have passed the State exams.' Not the most romantic engagement. The rest of my short stay we spent discussing our future, but first Ken suggested we go to the Petticoat Lane Market in the East End, as it was Sunday.

'Why there?'

'They have a jewellery area where there are often some lovely antique rings.' He grinned at me; 'I want to make it official!'

So we boarded the tube train and spent a while enjoying the unique experience of the famous London market. I marvelled at the 'barkers' selling their wares; some would have half a tea set balanced precariously along their outstretched arm calling out; 'see this amazing set I am offering you at half the price you would pay in Selfridges. What is the price you ask? It is worth ten pounds, but what am I offering you; not eight pounds, but just five pounds. It's a steal...' and pointing to a bystander... 'there you are madam, just for you, it is your lucky day.'

We made our way to a warehouse where the jewellery was displayed and certainly there was a lot of choice. I had been a little disappointed not to be bought a new ring, but as Ken explained, these were unique. I spent some time deliberating but finally settled on a fire opal surrounded by twelve small antique cut diamonds. As I held it up to the light small flames of red fire reflected and I wondered who had worn it before me, and pushed to the back of my mind the old wives' tale that opals were unlucky.

While I had been choosing, Ken had been looking at other rings.

'How about selecting your wedding ring too, Chris?'

I was not sure about a second-hand wedding ring, but agreed to look and finally chose an attractive gold and white gold plaited one which would offset the engagement ring.

'What about you, Ken?'

'Oh, men don't wear rings.'

'Some do these days.'

'Well I won't. It's effeminate.'

'It's a commitment.'

He smiled and shrugged. 'Isn't marrying you commitment enough?'

I did not argue as my rather Victorian upbringing had placed the man at the head of the family, but I was determined I was going to go on working as a nurse after we were married. I need not have worried when we discussed it with my future husband.

'That's fine. We need two incomes.' We were sitting in the seldom used 'front room' of Ken's home to have a little privacy. Ken grinned at me. 'Dad is offering 47 Tabley Road for us to buy from him. You know we used to live there till we moved out to Finchley but he kept it on. He's not charging us interest, but even so we will need to save as well as pay him back.'

Within three months, in May we were married.

I obviously displeased the Matron when I told her I was leaving to move to London to be married instead of carrying on with training, following my pass in the State exams, but by then my mind was firmly made up. My parents were not totally surprised but I knew my father was a little disappointed.

'Chrissie, this is a commitment for life. You are so young, just twenty-one and Ken is nine years older. Your personality is hardly formed and Ken is the man he will always be.' Prophetic words I was to remember many years later.

Momma and Pop came down to London from Yorkshire and my brother arrived from university to be best man. My maid of honour was my good friend Rosemary from school days and she stayed with me in my new home overnight, while Ken of course was at his parents' home; no sleeping together before marriage in those days.

The night before we sat and chatted and suddenly the enormity of what I was doing hit me. Did I really know this man I was about to tie myself to? He was almost a stranger. I looked at my friend in horror; 'Oh, Rosemary.; I don't know why I am marrying Ken.'

For a moment she sat stunned, then patted my hand. 'Just wedding nerves, Chrissie.' It was many years later she confided in me, that comment of mine made her doubly sure when she fell in love and married her husband.

We were married in St Luke's Anglican Church in Holloway to which the badminton club belonged, and which Ken had been attending. Uniquely we had a triumphal arch of badminton rackets held by the members. And although it rained, I was happy, looking forward to my new life as a wife in the busy city of London, the previous night's nerves pushed to the back of my mind.

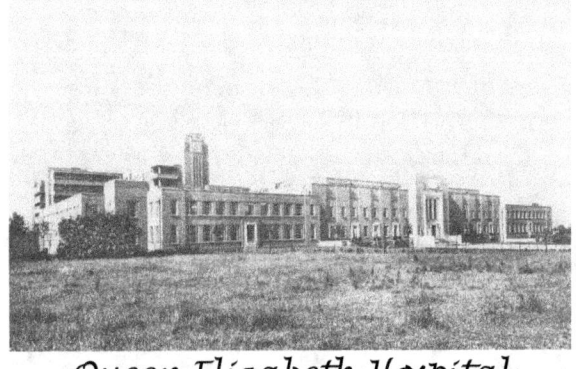

Queen Elizabeth Hospital
Circa 1950

The General Nursing Council for England and Wales

Record of Practical Instruction and Experience for the Certificate of General Nursing

Name of Student Nurse Christine Elizabeth Atkinson

Date of entry to training 6th January 1959

Index Number 82689

The items included in Section I of this Record are those in which a student nurse must have received instruction before entry to the Preliminary Examination although the student may not have attained proficiency. All items included in both Sections I and II should be covered before entry to the Final Examination.

Additional pages at the back of the Record refer to special experience, details of nursing care and should be filled in and signed by the Sister or Charge Nurse in the appropriate column.

The Sister or Charge Nurse, as the various items are taught, is requested to mark these in the appropriate column, one stroke (/) to signify that the student nurse has been instructed, but is not yet proficient, a X to signify that the student is proficient. The Sister or Charge Nurse will sign the Record in the appropriate column wherever a X is marked.

Further copies of this publication may be obtained from the offices of the Council. It may not be reprinted or reproduced either in whole or in part without the sanction of the Council.

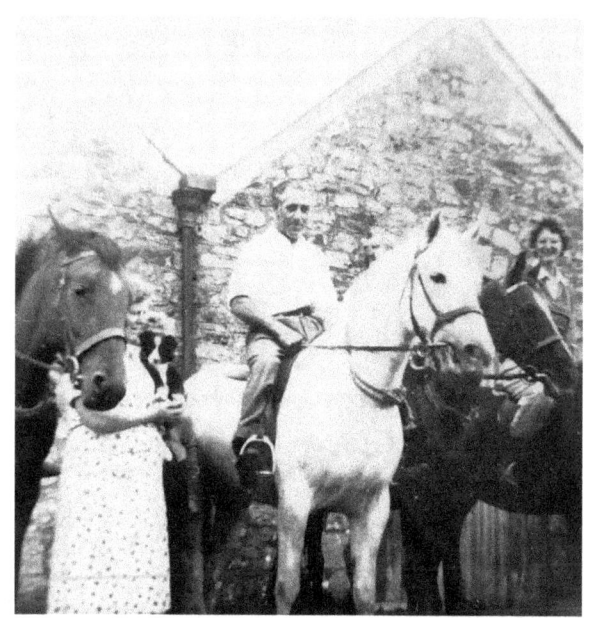

Our YHA pony trekking guide

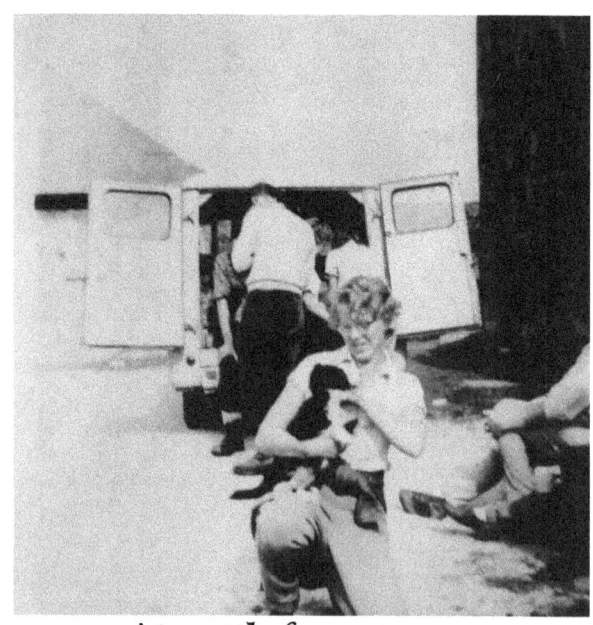

Me with farm puppy

PART 2
LONDON
1960-1966 and 1976

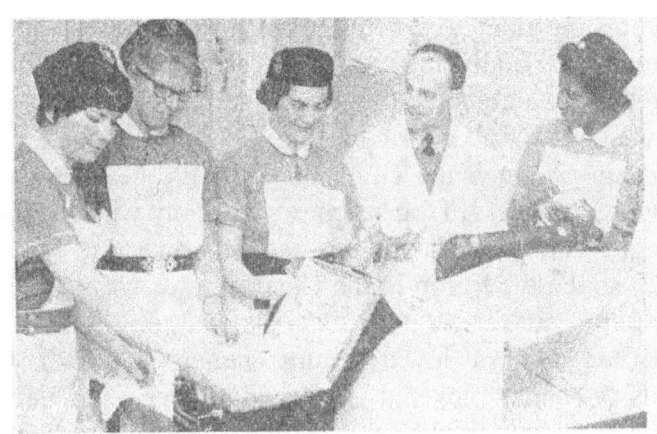

QIDN nurses preparing bags; I am second from left

2/1

We decided to spend our honeymoon on the tiny Feudal Island of Sark in the British Channel Isles. Having discovered this strange and unique place the previous year we both fell in love with the beautifully unspoiled countryside and relaxed lifestyle, so different from London.

We stayed at an old farmhouse run by a local couple who treated us like their own family, cooking wholesome food and spoiling us rotten. As it was warm May weather, the outside toilet was not a problem and the fact there were no cars added to the uniqueness. The Island, a high plateau, was only one mile wide by three and a half long so we found walking or cycling on the hired bikes no hardship although the climb down to the beaches gave enough exercise. All the beaches were stony with rounded shingle, except when the sea receded revealing golden sand, as the tidal drop in the Channel Isles was as much as twenty-four feet.

I had always loved natural countryside and the roadside banks covered with wildflowers and small wooded valleys bright green with new leaves enchanted me. Although a Londoner Ken had also learned to love the countryside too, as he had spent many happy hours walking on Hampstead Heath, an amazing open area of countryside in the northern part of the city. It is rambling and hilly, including ponds and recent and ancient woodlands. He also enjoyed swimming and it was on Sark he taught me in the icy Channel waters.

'I used to swim until quite late in the year, in the Highgate and Hampstead Ponds, you know.'

'Didn't it get cold; and what about your asthma?'

'It was good for that. If you keep it up, it helps the lungs to expand.'

So he patiently supported me in the water and taught me breast stroke, until I was confident to try on my own, though I never had the courage to get out of my depth.

We used to lie and dry on the beach if it was warm enough and talk about our future.

'I really want to be a district nurse, as you know, but there is a waiting list for the training.'

I looked up at the towering cliffs above and sighed. 'I wouldn't mind doing something a bit different for a while anyway.'

Ken looked at me with raised eyebrows. 'Thought you always wanted to be a nurse.'

'Yes of course, but I'd like to do something still connected to nursing, like dental assistant. I believe that is quite well paid.'

We were sad to leave the Island and both secretly had a fantasy of one day living there...but we felt it was just that; now I had to get a job. Ken was well paid as a junior manager in a large advertising firm in their publicity department, but as he explained:

'We need to save for the future, so I would like to put most of my salary towards that and live off what you earn.' Coming from a family where the man was the breadwinner and had the say where money was concerned, it seemed acceptable.

I felt I wanted to do my share.

We settled into our new home, and I became used to sharing a double bed with my husband and accepted there would be no flashes of light or bells ringing when we made love. I had read books and studied the male anatomy, more or less knowing what to expect on the wedding night. I had been looking forward to an exciting, though perhaps a little painful experience but on the morning after, my main thought was 'is that all there is to it. What is all the fuss about?' I began to believe the romances I had read as a teenager were greatly exaggerated.

Our new home, 47 Tabley Road, was a typical London terraced house, divided into two flats and a small bedsitting room. Entrance was up a couple of steps and through a door with a coloured glass fanlight. A narrow hall laid with lino gave access to the downstairs flat and a flight of steep stairs led to the rest of the house. There was a communal slot meter telephone on the wall, which was quite a luxury in those days.

The bottom flat was rented by a middle-aged couple and consisted of a kitchen, one bedroom and a sitting room, and they had joint use of the small back garden which was our responsibility. Up the flight of stairs from the communal front door and entrance hall, was our kitchen, and next to it the bathroom shared with an old lady in the bedsitting room on the top floor. The bathroom had a tub and gas water heater, and mercifully there was a separate toilet. Up another flight of stairs were our bedroom and a long, bay-windowed lounge. The final floor had the old lady's bedsit and another room the same size as the lounge without the bay window.

I was delighted with my new home and set about buying curtains and painting the lounge walls. I had been brought up by parents who were always on the move and so constantly 'doing up' their new home. I had at an early age been introduced to a paint brush. Most of the rooms in my new home were cream, not my favourite after living in the hospital environment where it seemed the standard colour, so I determined to change that as soon as possible.

The old lady in the bedsit, Mrs Thomas, was, I think lonely as she had a habit of listening for my return and trotting down to see if I was in the kitchen, often entering without knocking.

Until the one day when I was doing the washing.

Ken had bought me a twin tub washing machine and spin dryer for my wedding gift. To rinse the clothes it was necessary to transfer them from the washing machine to the separate spinner, which had a hole into which you inserted one end of a hose, with the other fixed to the tap. Care had to be taken not to push the end too far into the spinner, or the clothes caught onto it, dragging the end off the tap and swirling the hose around the room, spraying water in all directions. It so happened Mrs Thomas arrived one day just as this occurred and the poor woman was soaked as she opened the door.

After that she always knocked before entering.

For a few days after our return from Sark, I enjoyed settling in, but I needed to get a job.

This was to prove more difficult than I had anticipated. There were several advertisements for dental nurses in the papers, so I reasoned surely my qualification would be enough. The first three I approached wanted an experienced dental nurse; then I saw one for a secretary and dental assistant in Wimpole St, in the heart of London. This was the Harley Street of dentists, catering for the rich and famous. I decided to give it a try although it was only for two and a half days a week.

As I walked up the white scrubbed front steps I felt I had stepped back a century, and hoped I would not leave footprints on the pristine surface. The bell was an old fashioned brass pull chord, and the black clad woman who answered could have come out of a Dickens' novel.

'I have come to see Mr Mackintosh.'

'He is just with a patient, Miss. Do you have an appointment?'

'Er, yes; I mean I have come for the jo...position as secretary and assistant.'

She looked me up and down and sniffed. 'You are very young.'

'I am a highly qualified nurse. I am older than I look.'

She said nothing but told me to wait in the dark entrance hall with its luxurious carpet and hunting pictures on the wall. This was a far cry from any dentist I had attended.

Mr Macintosh did not look like a dentist either, more like a comfortable country squire, with his neat tweed jacket and a pipe in his hand. The voice was pure Oxbridge. 'Do come in Mrs Davies. Now tell me a little about yourself.'

'Well I am a trained nurse but admit I am not a dental nurse; but I am a quick learner.'

'Yes, but what is your background; family, schooling, that sort of thing?'

Looking around at the muted richness of the 'surgery' I realised this was not the traditional dentist. The treatment chair was leather bound and hardly seemed clinical, and few instruments were apparent. I later learned they were kept out of the way until needed, so the wealthy patients would not be upset by their sight on arrival. It was obvious Mr Macintosh was seeking an assistant with the proper background, so I put on my best voice, grateful that I had lost my Yorkshire accent with my parents' many moves about the country.

'I went to Grammar School in Stratford-on-Avon, where I lived most of my schooling years and where my father was the Customs and Excise officer.'(May I be forgiven for my pretension.) 'We were fortunate to attend the theatre on many occasions, seeing some of the most famous actors and actresses, you know; Peggy Ashcroft, Laurence Olivier, Vivien Leigh, and so on.'

'Well that is satisfactory. You see, we have several titled patients and they expect a certain degree of, shall I say cosseting. You will be able to pick up the rest. Can you type and do you know how to develop x-rays?'

I thought of my father's old typewriter and how I had tried to teach myself touch typing, without much success and my brother's hobby of printing his photos, which I had watched.

'Well, yes I can do a little,'

'It will be just a few appointment reminders and so on and x-rays to develop. So when can you start?'

'You mean I have the job?'

2/2

It seemed the previous assistant had left to get married, and Mr Macintosh needed me as soon as I was free. So I agreed to start the next day.

When I announced my success, Ken was not as impressed as I would have liked. 'It's only two and a half days a week, though, Chris.'

'Well... I'll get another for the rest of the week. I shall be happy to have weekends off after all these years.'

I decided not to look for anything else until I became used to this new career, reasoning I would then be able to say I was experienced. It certainly was very different from working in a hospital and the patients reminded me a little of the time I was in the private hospital ward. Several were titled and all were wealthy expecting preferential treatment. I soon discovered the difference between the *'nouveaux riche'* and the genuine aristocracy. The former who had gained their wealth recently by business, treated me like a servant, while I believe many of the others, the '*Aristocracy*' saw me as a professional person; not talking down to me, or just ignoring me.

Mr Mackintosh was a gentleman and treated his patients with respect, but also firmly when needed. I found pain was no discriminator, and the wealthy were as scared of dental work as we lesser mortals. A large proportion of the work involved taking impressions for dentures, and I soon learned how to mix the thick paste used, then to label them properly and deliver the imprint to the technician on the lower floor. Then when the dentures were ready, I had to collect and bring them for Mr Mackintosh for a patient's fitting. I was always a little anxious not to drop them on the way up the stairs.

I was taught how to develop the x-rays which were taken for most patients. The 'laboratory' was a converted deep cupboard which was set in the wooden panelling which surrounded most of the room. I am slightly claustrophobic and did not take too happily to shutting myself into the confined dark cubbyhole which had been set up with all the paraphernalia needed. There was a red light, which helped a little. I soon learned to mix the chemicals and soak the small plates, watching anxiously as the x-rays developed, then hanging them up to dry with little clips and making sure I had the right patient's name on them.

My other responsibilities were mixing the fillings when requested and handing the appropriate instruments to Mr Mackintosh. My theatre experience had taught me to observe what a particular person liked to use and have the right equipment ready. I think Mr Mackintosh was pleased with my observation, as sometimes he would start to ask for an implement just as I was about to pass it to him.

Letter writing was another duty but one I laboured over, and I often found myself staying behind after Mr Mackintosh had left, trying to get it right.

I quite enjoyed the novelty of the work, and some of the patients were interesting if a little eccentric. One in particular insisted on bringing in a box of sticky sweet cakes called Rum Babas whenever she visited. As she was being fitted with dentures which necessitated several visits, this was a regular occasion. Neither the dentist nor I liked these cakes and were hard put to look delighted when yet another box from Selfridges arrived. The elderly lady was so keen to give us our treat; we had not the heart to refuse. I did wonder if she herself liked to indulge and her own teeth had suffered as a consequence.

After a couple of weeks, and to satisfy Ken's insistence, I explored the *'situations vacant'* in the papers to supplement my part time work. I decided I would look for another dental post, feeling confident I had enough experience now.

'Position offered for a Registered Nurse to assist dentist.' The advert seemed made for me; the only problem, it was the other side of London in the East End.

I studied the underground map and discovered I could use the Bakerloo line with just a short walk each end, so made an appointment for an interview.

This could not have been more different from my other job and more what I had expected of a dental surgery. So was the dentist Paul Levi, who looked the quintessential Jew which he was; a neat man, with classic long nose and bright dark eyes which missed nothing. He got straight to the point as soon as I had introduced myself.

'Many of my patients have had little or no dental treatment in their lives. When they come to me there is nothing I can do but remove several, sometimes all, of their teeth. They would never be persuaded to come here more than once, so it is all I can do for them. To do this I need to give a general anaesthetic by intravenous injection.' He looked me up and down. 'I will need to see proof of your qualification, as I need to have an SRN in attendance.'

I said I would bring proof, but then added, 'However I can only work two and a half days a week, as I have a part time dental position elsewhere.' For some reason I hesitated to say where I was already working; the difference between Mr Mackintosh's patients and those I would see here were poles apart, but Mr Levi did not seem to be interested. He thought for a moment, then shrugged.

'That will be alright I suppose. My wife can assist with the lighter work. I expect you will want a higher wage as an SRN? What are you earning now?'

I named my hourly rate, which was quite good for the sort of work I was doing. For a moment I thought I was going to be rejected, then Mr Levi nodded and we discussed days and times. My only concern was the day I worked half a day in Wimpole Street and had to travel across London for the afternoon. On that day, Mr Levi had a late clinic which meant I did not need to arrive until two o'clock.

I was now working five days a week, with a long day on Wednesdays. I would be earning a good wage; more than I had done so far. As a student there had been little payment, for we were being trained and had board and lodging included.

The work in the East End could not have been more different from that in Wimpole Street. Most of the patients were Cockneys from the streets around, and the rooms were a traditional clinical setup with tilting chair and that peculiar aroma of disinfectant, mouthwash and a slight hint of oil of cloves.

My boss was very different too.

There was no time for chatting or indulging in sticky cakes; work was the keyword. We were there to offer treatment swiftly and as efficiently as possible. I quite enjoyed the challenge, and it reminded me a little of my operating theatre times, as it was my duty particularly to look after people while they were under anaesthetic and afterwards. Mr Levy preferred to choose his own instruments...which were mostly various forceps for extractions. There was a small recovery room at the back, and I was to supervise patients returning to consciousness and make sure they did not choke, and of course reassure them. It must have been traumatic, especially for the many young people, to wake up suddenly to an empty and bloody mouth.

The weeks passed and I enjoyed being at home at weekends. Ken was usually there too, though sometimes had duties at the Youth Club, especially on Saturday night. I often went with him and really enjoyed playing badminton. At other times we would take our bikes out towards Epping Forest, cycling down canal towpaths to reach this lovely unspoiled area.

One day in late spring Ken suggested a novel idea for a Youth Club outing.

'You know, Chris, some of these youngsters have seldom been out of London and I bet they have never seen the midsummer sunrise in the country.'

'What do you have in mind?'

'I'd like to take them to Box Hill in Surrey on midsummer night and watch the sun rise.'

'How would we get there?'

'We can all take a bus, but first I think you and I should take a trip out on our bikes next weekend. We can cycle down the towpaths of some of the canals.'

It sounded a fun idea, so I agreed.

2/3

Ken and I enjoyed our trip out by bike. We were used to rough riding and managed to get to the very top of Box Hill where Ken said we would have the best view of the rising sun on Midsummer Day. Way below spread the Surrey Downs and it seemed amazing we were only nineteen miles south of the big city of London. I revelled in the green growing smells, wildflowers and shading trees. Although we often went to Hampstead Heath and Highgate in London itself, somehow it did not feel like proper countryside. You could always hear the muted traffic noise with the occasional ambulance or police siren in the distance and the vegetation seemed dusty and tired. Here you could look down at the small settlements and follow the glint of sunlight reflected from a windscreen as a tiny car made its way through the country lanes. Lazy cattle grazed in the brilliantly green fields, and the only sounds were the rustle of leaves and birdsong.

It was still only the beginning of June, so we had to wait for the longest day around the twenty first, so we had a few weeks of work before the outing. I had settled into my two jobs, but realised I really preferred 'proper nursing.' I had applied to the Queens Institute of District Nursing but there was no vacancy yet, and I would need to take a three month training first in any case. Once I had mastered the routines in dental nursing, there was little challenge, but one day something occurred to cause a distraction.

It was on one of my East End days while I was taking a lunch break; I heard the unmistakable screech of brakes, a scream and then a babble of voices across the road from the surgery. I went outside to see an elderly woman lying on the road by the curb, and so rushed over to see if I could help. She was a quintessential 'Eastender', with hair in curlers and was wrapped in an all over apron; wiry and tough looking. I asked what had happened and one of the bystanders explained.

'Her was goin' ter step off the curb like, and that there van'...he pointed to a delivery van with *'Walkers' Vegetables; speedy delivery straight from Covent Garden,'* blazoned on the side, "'ee backed into er, didn't ee?' The young driver with a worried expression was standing by the open drivers' door. 'Didn't give me no chance, did she? Just stepped off wivout lookin.' Adding in a mutter *'silly old bat'*

I knelt down as the woman complained; 'Oo me legs, me legs.' I looked up and someone said they had phoned 999, so I just tried to calm her and keep her comfortable. I tried to examine her but she kept pushing my hand away with a 'wat yer doin?'. I could see no obvious injury but I realised she could have internal trauma so just said; 'Just you lie there, try not to move.'

All went well until an ambulance arrived, sirens blaring.

The woman suddenly sat up and stared at the two ambulance men as they climbed out of the vehicle. She then staggered to her feet, shook herself and declared; 'I'm not going in that bleedin' ambulance.' Spun on her heel and pushed her way through the gathering crowd. I could only hope she had not been bruised but there was nothing I could do to help in any case.

That, and my interacting with the youth club members, who were mostly from a deprived background, made me realised what a privileged background I had experienced. I realised once I was able to work among them as a district nurse, I would have a whole new view of how other people lived in this big city.

I wondered how our youngsters would react to a trip out in the country.

Soon Midsummer Day approached and so on the next club day Ken said he had an announcement to make, while we were all taking a break from our vigorous games of badminton.

'You probably know it will soon be Midsummer Day. Does anyone know anything special about that?'

'Do they dance round a pole or something?'

Ken laughed; 'No, that's *Mayday*. I'll tell you: it's the longest time of daylight in the year, and the sun hardly sets before it rises again at about four in the morning. It is quite amazing, and especially when you can see it from a place like 'Box Hill.'

They silently watched Ken, so he continued. 'We thought you'd like a trip out there and see for yourselves. We can take a sort of picnic and make an outing of it. What d'you say?'

At the idea of a trip most of the youngsters became enthusiastic. I supposed they did not have many outings.

The day before Midsummer Day, we met as agreed to board the bus which would take us most of the way, with a change to a local one at the end. It was fine weather, though not particularly warm. As we collected together at the base of Box Hill I looked round at the clothes of the young people. We had suggested they wore strong shoes and protective clothing, but I realised many did not have other than their every-day clothes. Most of the girls had flimsy dresses and cardigans and lightweight shoes. The boys were better clad, with heavier shoes and work trousers. I kicked myself for not thinking ahead. Maybe we could have supplied something from second hand shops. I was certainly glad of my stout walking boots as there had been some rain and it was quite muddy.

We set off and Ken and the older boys helped the girls over styles and through farm gates until we reached the base of the hill. It was easier going then as there were proper paths to follow.

Everyone had been asked to bring a picnic and something to drink and I had included a first aid kit, for which I was going to be grateful; there were several bramble scratches and abrasions before the day was over. We had also packed extra food as I was not sure if they all would be able to bring enough for themselves. At least I had thought ahead for that.

Eventually we arrived, hot and sweating at a flattened area looking out to the eastern plains. There was a natural hollow shaded by trees behind us and we were relieved to settle down and eat our sandwiches. My admiration for these rough kids grew as those who had brought food gladly shared with those who had little. I was reminded of the Bible story of the boy with loaves and fishes, whose food fed thousands. I had always thought it was a story of people being shamed into sharing what they had secretly brought to eat themselves, after seeing the generosity of the young boy; which in itself was a miracle.

When we had all eaten our fill, there was still a little left for our breakfast. As the light faded...it never really became black night...we sat around and sang songs, watching the glow from London a long away on the horizon, until one by one, we settled down for the few hours before the sun would appear again at about four a.m.

I was pretty tired and lay down under a tree but felt itchy and did not really sleep. It was only when Ken called us all awake, I realised why I had been restless.

I had lain on an ants' nest.

'Chris, your eye is all swollen.' I could hardly see Ken, and realised I had been bitten on my eyelid; I felt such an idiot.

I had packed a tube of antihistamine cream and had not expected to need it for myself, but there was no time for self-pity, as the eastern sky was beginning to lighten. Slowly a bright pinpoint appeared, and we watched spellbound as gradually the orange sun slid up over the horizon, sending shafts of golden light through the countryside. It picked out the windows of a farmhouse with a quick diamond glint then sent long shadows creeping over fields, waking a cockerel whose strident crow we could hear faintly in the still air. Our usually noisy youngsters were silent, whether from tiredness or awe I was not sure, but hoped we had given some pleasant memory to be stored away for their future.

After eating the food we had left and waiting till full light, we made our weary way home. It seemed quicker returning, and as we walked I asked one young girl if she had enjoyed the adventure. She thought for a moment then shook her head.

'It's awright for them that lives there, but lor, I'd not know what to do with all that there space, Mrs Chris,'

2/4

As the weeks passed, I realised I was missing 'real' nursing, and as there was still no vacancy for the Queen's Institute training, I began to read the *'situations vacant'* in the papers again, and felt it was only fair to warn my two employers. I did feel a little mean in letting them down.

Mr Macintosh was not surprised but a little disappointed.

'I didn't really think your heart was in it, Christine, but the patients liked you. You have a way with people.' He sighed and asked, 'Can you work the month out? I will have to advertise again.'

Mr Levi was abrupt as usual, just shrugged and paying me a week in advance, said,

'You might as well finish today, then.'

That was a bit of a shock as we needed the income to pay off the loan on our house. Ken's father had kindly not charged us interest, but of course we had to repay the 6,000 pounds for the property on a regular basis. The rent from the flats helped with repayments but housekeeping mostly came out of my earnings. I never knew what Ken earned, and anyway he was saving it for 'contingencies and a rainy day' as he put it.

'Well, this is one of them,' I complained when I told him of my decision.

'You'll get another job soon, Chris. They are always crying out for nurses.'

He was right. It was not long before I applied and was offered a position more to my liking. The Marie Curie Hospital in Hampstead specialised in radium implantations for women with uterine cervical cancer and my work would mostly be in the theatre and the outpatients' department. I discovered the small hospital had been opened in 1929 and the famous scientist, Marie Currie, who had discovered Radium was very interested in the treatment there, allowing her name to be used. The original building had suffered in bombing raids in the Second World War, and the hospital was now housed in a temporary building while plans were made for a new hospital on the old site. The present location was in a converted disused hall and was a little cramped. There were a basic operating theatre, a pre-med room and small recovery ward similar to those attached to the casualty ward in the Queen Elizabeth hospital in Birmingham, but the equipment was a little dated.

It was my job to load the radium needles onto special forceps and hand them to the surgeon who then inserted them into the uterine cervix of the anesthetised patient. I was exposed to radiation and had to wear a heavy lead-impregnated apron and always have on my special badge which would record how much radiation I had received.

It was also my duty to pack and sterilise the drums in which were packed the dressings used during the operations.

Housed in the basement in what I think had been a coal bunker, the ancient autoclave had a mind of its own. After packing the round metal drums and making sure the ventilation holes around the sides were open so the steam could penetrate, I had to fix down the locks on the autoclave's lid. A large dial showed the pressure, and it was necessary to make sure the needle did not spin round onto the red zone, or the whole thing was in danger of exploding. Sometimes the needle stuck, and had to be thumped hard when it did, in order to get an accurate reading. When the necessary time had elapsed, pressure was released and the drums allowed to cool, then they were pulled out using a special hook, the slats in the drums closed and then they all were taken back up to the theatre.

I enjoyed the work, though it became a little repetitive after a while. I had the most interest in the outpatients' department, as we saw women as a follow up who had attended the Royal Free Hospital with breast cancer treatment. It was wonderful to realise our lecturers were not entirely correct in indicting a high mortality rate from this common malady. Women came after many years of freedom from cancer, and not showing any signs of recurrence, or secondary cancers.

Periodically we had our badges checked to record the amount of radiation we had been exposed to and after a couple of months I was warned my reading was becoming rather high. As I wanted to have a family some time and was afraid this might affect my fertility, I decided the best choice would be to leave as soon as I could.

I was out of work once more and still there was no good news from the Queen's Institute of District Nursing, so I was back studying the *'situations vacant'* yet again.'

I was becoming a little despondent and Ken could see I was tired of the several work changes and surprised me one evening after he had returned home. He pulled a leaflet from his pocket, and I could see it had the green triangle of the Youth Hostel Association badge on the front.

'How would you like to go to Italy for a holiday?'

It was just what I needed to cheer me and soon we were planning to meet the YHA guide who would escort the dozen or so of us, first to Rome, then the Island of Sardinia. Ken and I had current passports and so were all set to go in a month's time, having had instructions about what to pack.

'Remember you will have to carry your own belongings, so I suggest a rucksack is the best bet.' I had bought an Army surplus kaki knapsack which I had used for Youth Hostelling in previous holidays, so I decided that would be my best bet, especially as I had proudly sewn various badges from different Hostels onto it.

I realised I would need to have some employment in the meantime and was fortunate to be engaged to work in the outpatients' department of the Whittington Hospital, St Mary's wing in Holloway, which was in walking distance from our home. I had made sure my two-week holiday would be honoured, of course, and fortunately this was not a problem as they were short of qualified staff.

I had always enjoyed the variety of outpatients, and soon I was taught to take blood samples from patients, which did not worry me despite my slight sensitivity to the sight of blood. I became quite adept at locating the veins in the patient's arm, though I learned it was advisable to lie my patients down before beginning. Soon after I had taken over the blood clinic a young *'macho'* type arrived, and I sat him down on the chair. I turned round to read the request form and select the specimen bottles and then swung round with the syringe and needle in my hand. I was just in time to see my patient blanch and slide to the floor in a dead faint.

The outpatients' department was mostly routine, but it had its moments. Patients had to sit on a chair by reception to be admitted, and one day I walked by catching an almost overpowering whiff of 'Old Spice', one of my favourite men's aftershaves. Thinking there might be an attractive young man there, I peeped over to see an elderly man with a shining bald head from which waves of 'Old Spice' were filling the waiting room. Ever after that perfume reminded me of that man and his shiny head.

One day the sister called me into her office.

'Davies, I think you said you had some theatre experience? We have a small minor ops theatre here; just removal of cysts and lumps under local, mostly: occasionally a baby for a routine circumcision. Would you like to take it on?'

I was delighted and soon organised the young newly qualified doctors who came to operate, and as the sister indicated, it was mostly routine procedures, but I was horrified when I observed a circumcision for the first time. After the baby had a light general anaesthetic, the surgeon pulled the foreskin over the end of the baby's little penis, clamped the tissue with a pair of forceps and sliced with a scalpel. One slip and there would be irreparable damage. For a while a junior Registrar attended to this operation, but eventually it was passed on to the newly qualified young doctors who had me watching anxiously. One such seemed to be very unsure of himself, and as he was about to clamp the end of the little mite's penis, I had to intervene.

'Excuse me doctor, but with all due respect, have you done this before?'

'Erm, well no, not really, nurse.'

I had no recourse but to show him how and ended up doing it myself as he was so clumsy. I hoped to goodness he was not planning to take up surgery.

My month in the outpatients' department passed quickly, and soon we were on our way to Italy: my first real trip overseas.

2/5

I found the holiday exciting from the beginning. We were due to meet the leader and the rest of the party at Victoria Station and Ken explained what would happen. He loved train travel and had studied our whole trip.

'We will be on what they call the *"Night Ferry,"* which is loaded onto the ship complete at Dover...'

'You mean the carriages are put onto the ferry with us inside?'

'Um, I don't think so. I assume we re-board the carriages on the ferry boat. Anyway, we sleep in special bunks and travel through Europe on the same train.'

'So we won't see the countryside at all?'

'Not unless you stay awake.'

'I jolly well will, then. I don't want to miss anything.'

Ken laughed, but I was determined to stay awake. I knew we would be passing through France and then Switzerland before making our way to Rome.

Tony our guide was easy to locate as he was holding up a large YHA sign, and was surrounded by several other young people, dressed casually as we were and with rucksacks of varying sizes piled to one side. I was surprised to see some large backpacks and wondered what on earth they contained. I had packed what I thought I might need for ten days, but only had one changes of clothes as well as a well-equipped first aid kit, realising I would have to carry everything myself.

There were four women and six men already waiting and I was sure you could pick out Youth Hostellers from other travellers. We all wore casual and serviceable skirts or, for the men, shorts or trousers. A couple of the women wore lipstick, as did I but no other makeup. I suppose we looked a drab bunch when you compared us with the holiday clothing of other people arriving to board the train. I even saw a woman carrying a pillow.

Our leader looked rather impatient as we awaited the final couple, and he kept glancing at his watch. The last two arrived and Tony said it was time to board the train as it was now almost nine in the evening but I was too excited to feel tired as the train sped through the summer countryside.

Our adventure had begun.

It was June and so the fields, villages and woodlands were still bathed in late evening golden light as we sped on our way to Dover. All too soon we arrived at the docks and were shepherded through the embarkation process. It was a relief to have someone who knew exactly what to do and where to go. At first when I knew we were going to have a guide, I was not too keen on the idea of being moved around like a herd of cattle as I had seen in Stratford on Avon, among the visitors there. The guide would be holding a placard or umbrella as people trotted behind like a pied piper and his entourage.

The ferry we boarded was like the one we had used on our visits to the Channel Isles, and I felt quite at home, and we all enjoyed wandering around and exploring, but Tony asked us all to collect at a particular point when the disembarking call was made. At last we arrived in France and boarded the train again which was waiting at the platform, to locate our sleeping compartments. It all was so well organised.

We were sharing a cabin with another couple, and I was not too happy about that, wondering how they would cope with Ken's snoring. His asthma and breathing problems sometimes produced noises more appropriate to the farmyard, but I had become used to it, using earplugs which were moderately effective. In fact there was a competition with the other man, so had I wished to sleep it would have been difficult. I was happy at first to lie with my head towards the window, pulling the blind aside to watch our progress through the outskirts of Paris. I briefly saw the Eifel tower outlined against spotlights, and then the backs of many tenement buildings looking peculiarly French, with strings of onions and lines of washing hanging out of casement windows.

I witnessed little flashes of other peoples' lives as we sped by: a young couple kissing by the open window; a little girl fighting with an older boy who was pulling at her teddy; an older couple leaning on a small balcony with glasses of wine in their hands, and I amused myself with making up stories to go with those little flashes. The young couple were newly married and very much in love: the teddy had belonged to the little boy, but now it was his sister's and he wanted it back: the older couple had been lovers and separated, now re-united and sharing their past lives.

Gradually the buildings gave way to country scenes; fields cut for hay; pretty villages of thatched or tiled roofed cottages and several tumbling streams and rivers. Eventually the swaying of the carriage and regular clacking of the rails won, and I slipped into a fitful sleep, to be woken with a start as we stopped at the border with Switzerland.

Here again we were fortunate as Tony had taken charge of our passports and attended to the Customs officers and could speak fluent French. Soon we were on our way, but I was wide awake and peeped through my window again, to delight in shadowy snow-clad mountains of the Swizz Alps and picturesque villages straight out of travel brochures.

By the time we crossed over the Italian border I was very sleepy and must have dozed as the next thing I heard was Tony sliding back the door and warning us to be ready to arrive in about ten minutes. Dozy and half asleep we collected on the platform of Rome's Termini Station wondering how soon we could go to the Youth Hostel where we were to spend four nights.

'You will find Youth Hostelling in Europe a little different, but I am sure you will enjoy it just the same.' Tony hesitated a moment. 'We have some trips organised, particularly to the catacombs, but you will have time on your own, but I would suggest you keep in groups of at least two.' He looked a little serious. 'There have been a few demonstrations against the Germans and as some of you are fair haired, remember the Italian for *'English'* is *'Inglese.'* If anyone accosts you just point to yourself and say *'Inglese!* Now normally we can't go to the Hostel till three this afternoon, but I have arranged an early sign in as I guess some of you might want a nap. Many people here do have a siesta anyway.'

With that he herded his sleepy group across busy roadways and down narrow streets until we arrived at a rambling old building with a covered extended pergola type patio in the front.

'That's the dining area; just hope it doesn't rain.' Tony looked up at the billowing clouds and laughed. 'After we have checked in you can have a few hours resting or sorting yourselves or go and explore. Be back here at seven tonight; we go to a *"Trattoria"* for your first taste of Italian food. You must try the drink *"Asti-Spumante".'*

Ken and I had enjoyed Italian food in London so this was going to be a test to see how authentic it all was in comparison. First, we left our packs in the dormitories (unfortunately separated male and female; no married quarters here!) and decided we did not wish to miss anything, so joined a few others in our first exploration. Ken had managed to get a map of Rome so we hoped we would not get lost.

Our group of six included a couple of very fair-haired brothers from Yorkshire, Bill and Barney. I secretly nicknamed them *"Bill and Ben the Flowerpot men"* from the children's TV programme, as one would often answer for the other. With their thick North Country accents they were almost like a comedy act and I was looking forward to their company during our short holiday. Our Teutonic appearance attracted the attention when we arrived at a wide road, and we discovered a demonstration in progress against Germany. We were relieved to be able to point to ourselves and shout *"Inglese! Inglese! English!"* as Tony had wisely advised us. Even so we had some less than friendly glances, so a little shaken we all decided to return to the Youth hostel and I for one was grateful for Ken's map. The rest of the afternoon I spent lazing in the sun as the clouds had disappeared, and writing post cards to my brother and parents.

In the evening our trip out for the meal was interesting but I was too tired to join in with much merrymaking, though the bubbly *Asti spumante* went down well.

2/6

After a good nights' sleep, we met in the dining area, sitting at long trestle tables and enjoying large bowl-like cups of strong black coffee and delicious crispy rolls with rather insipid jam. I sat with Ken and it seemed strange not to have spent the night with him; the first since we were married.

'Did you sleep OK?' I would have been surprised if Ken hadn't as he was able to 'kip' as he put it, anywhere.

'Yes thanks; and you?'

I nodded and he held up the roll he was eating. 'I'm going to miss my *"All bran"* and fresh fruit, though.' He was a man of habit.

'Well, you know what they say, *"When in Rome, do as the Romans".'*

We were soon called to group together by Tony as he told us about the day's activity he had planned.

'I thought today we could have a walk around to see the sights. We aren't far from the Coliseum and on the way we can look at the Victor Emmanuel Monument. He was the first King of a united Italy, and this building was erected on what was called Capitoline Hill and has come to symbolise the nations' patriotism. We will then walk to the Trevi fountain, which is one of the oldest water sources in Rome as it dates to about the 19th century BC.' He smiled; 'that's your history lesson for today but remember to have a few coins handy. I suppose you know the tradition, if you throw coins into the fountain, you will return one day?'

One of the party, a pretty dark haired girl, laughed and said, 'I heard one coin was to return; two you will fall in love and three, you would return and marry your lover?' She smiled sweetly at the young man by her side, who looked a little alarmed. Tony grinned again and raised his eyebrows; 'Who knows?'

We set off and I was glad I had put on my floppy sunhat and rubbed suntan cream on my arms, as the sun was very hot, although I could see huge billowing clouds appearing again. I was also pleased I was pretty fit from the cycling Ken and I had been used to, as the walk was quite extensive. I had seen photos in travel magazines of the Coliseum but was a little surprised when we finally arrived. It was bigger than I had expected, and I was interested to see it was quite well preserved. The rows of stone seats were all intact and below we explored the areas where the gladiators would have been housed. If you closed your eyes, it was not hard to imagine the roar of the crowds and smell the sweat and sawdust.

The Trevi Fountain was beautiful, but to my mind spoiled by all the tourists throwing coins over their shoulders. I would like to have been there at night, with the sound of tumbling water and the muted light of the streetlamps.

I think we were all relieved to return to the Hostel in the late afternoon. I could quite see why locals thought it a good idea to have a lie down in the middle of the day.

The next, out final day in Rome, Tony called us all together again and told us we were going to visit the Roman Catacombs which were about a fifteen-minute drive away. I admit I was not too keen, with my tendency to claustrophobia, but decided to give it a go. A small minibus collected us and as we sped through the seemingly chaotic traffic, I was glad I was not a district nurse in Rome. I said as much to Tony as he was sitting just in front of us.

'I was meaning to say, Chris; glad to have a trained nurse with us, just in case.' Ken raised his eyebrows but said nothing and I knew he sometimes found it embarrassing when people asked my advice about medical matters. He once said, after that had happened at a party.

'They wouldn't ask a plumber or solicitor for advice for free, would they?' But I did not mind; I was proud of my profession.

As we drove along, the clouds had been gathering again and as we arrived, the first large spots of rain landed, sending up puffs of dust in the road. Tony turned round and told us we were approaching the hidden *Catacombs of Domitilla* created by the early Romans as burial was not allowed inside the city.

'These Catacombs are a Christian cemetery named after the Domitilla family. You will see examples of artwork on the walls and there are over 26,000 tombs, situated over sixteen metres underground.' He looked out at the new steady rain: 'it's the best thing to be doing now. I suggest we run for it; the rain is quite warm, so don't worry you'll soon dry out.'

I was becoming increasingly uncomfortable with the thought of being that far underground but when we arrived, everything was quite well illuminated, and I did find it quite interesting. By the time we found our way back to the entrance I was relieved to approach daylight again, although it was to see torrential rain and a waterlogged road.

'No chance of getting the minibus through this; we'll just have to walk it.'

And so we did.

The water was warm as was the rain and several of us pranced through it singing at the top of our voices; the locals must have thought us mad. It was only afterwards Tony told us several manhole covers had been pushed up by the flood and he had worries we might have disappeared down one of them. My other concern was my skirt and blouse set was soaking and we were moving on the next day. I had to pack those and all I had was my reserve outfit for the rest of the holiday and I sadly realised I had been a little too economical with my packing.

The next day dawned as if there had been no rain as we made our way to Porto Civitavecchia some fifty miles from Rome, again taken by the small minibus. I was really enjoying the excitement of travel and decided to try to persuade Ken to take more holidays abroad. In the meantime we boarded the small ferry for the ride to Cagliari in the south of the island. It was really packed with people, and many seemed to be visitors. I was a little surprised as I knew until quite recently the island had a Malaria problem due to the many mosquitoes. By the intervention of the American Rockefeller Foundation just after the Second World War, extensive spraying of DDT had mainly controlled this, but I had not realised it was becoming so popular. By the sound of the conversations, I realised most of the people were Italian. All the signs and notices were also in Italian and I wished I had learned a little before starting this holiday. I spoke reasonable French, as it had been one of my best subjects at school and had thought the languages similar. Which they were not as I was to discover when I went to the toilet, trying to decide if I should use that marked *Signora* or *Signor,* and being totally bemused as each seemed to be used equally by either sex.

On arrival we made our way to the Youth Hostel housed in an old building, but we were soon off again exploring. It was a picturesque old city, the Capital of Sardinia with colourful terraced buildings at the harbour and the old part, the Citadel, rising on the hills beyond.

The next day, off we went again in a rickety old bus, up into the mountains. I remembered stories of bandits still inhabiting these areas and I think we were all relived to arrive at our destination, a lovely village which seemed far removed from modern life. Nearly everyone was dressed in the tradition costume, and obviously they were unused to visitors. We were beckoned by young women to visit and sample local cooking, as we wandered round the narrow steep lanes.

We kept together, as Tony said it would be easy to get lost and as we sat in the shade of a tree in a small square for a rest, we could hear music and singing. Tony stood up and called us to watch as a procession entered. 'A wedding; what luck...but be careful; no photos as they still believe cameras are the *"evil eye"* and could take offense.' Spellbound we watched as the young couple in full costume walked the area of the square followed by their colourful attendants, finally disappearing down a steep flight of stairs. It was magic and set the tone for our stay in Sardinia. I for one was sad when we returned to the mainland on our way back to London and so-called civilisation.

2/7

The trip home was a bit of an anti-climax as returns often are, but at least it was in daylight and we could enjoy the Swiss countryside. The little villages we had passed during the outward trip had a less romantic appearance now, especially as the rain had travelled north, but the snow-clad mountains to my mind were more mysterious, as they drifted in and out of misty rain, suddenly appearing like an iceberg in a rain-washed sea.

All too soon we were back in London, to drizzle and cold temperatures, but I had a pleasant surprise waiting.

On the hall table among the mail our tenants had kindly placed for us, was one from the Queens' Institute of District Nursing. Unable to wait, I sat on the bottom step leading up to our flat, much to Ken's amusement, and tore open the envelope.

I waved it at him; 'At last I can start my training in a month as long as I pass the interview.'

'It's what you wanted. Just hope it isn't a disappointment, and you still have to pass the interview.'

I was too happy to be annoyed with Ken's aptitude to look on the negative side. I was beginning to realise he was a 'cup half empty' type while I admitted I was more of a cup overflowing type, but I still had hopes of changing my husband's attitude in those early days.

The only unpleasant part was having to tell the outpatients' department I would be leaving as I hoped to become a district nurse if I passed the interview, but they took it in good part.

'You're lucky, Christine, they don't take many new nurses on. Let me know how the interview goes and we can work out your leaving date. You didn't sign a contract so I suppose a week's notice will be sufficient.' The charge sister looked out at the Autumn rain, 'though I don't envy you cycling round in this if they do take you on.'

The District Nursing Headquarters were in the London district of Canonbury, and I attended my interview with some trepidation. Supposing Ken had been right, and I failed; what would I do then? The sister in charge who was examining me reminded me a little of our tutor at the training school, but she was far more amenable.

'Why do you want to be a district nurse, Mrs Davies?'

'I like people and I think they are more in need of genuine help in their own homes.' I knew it sounded trite, but it was how I felt.

'That is true, but idealistic. How will you deal with the lack of sanitation; cluttered and overpopulated homes?' She shook her head with a rueful smile, 'You'll find flats in the three or four stories of the tenements often lead onto an open landing exposed to the elements and with a communal lavatory, usually overflowing, at each end. lifts seldom work, smelling as if used as an addition toilet.'

'I will learn.'

She looked at me for a moment, then surprised me by saying, 'I understand you are not long married. Do you plan a family?'

I bridled a little at that, but then realised it probably was important. Ken and I had discussed this before we married and agreed we would wait a few years, both thinking it would be a good idea to have two children close together.

'We don't plan a family yet.'

For a moment she tapped the paper in front of her with a 'Biro' then seemed to make up her mind, looking up and smiling.

'Do you have a bicycle, Mrs Davies, or will you be walking?' It was a moment before I realised she had said 'will,' so took a chance. 'Does that mean I am accepted?'

The sister nodded and smiled again. 'You will have a trial and then a small exam. How soon can you start? We do need some younger nurses as several are leaving soon.' I explained my present situation and we made an appointment for two weeks' time for me to attend the headquarters to be shown the procedures and to discuss the area I would be covering.

I had enjoyed my short stay at the outpatients' department and in particular my stint running the minor ops theatre and consoled myself with the knowledge of perhaps saving a few babies from complications from botched circumcisions. Now at last I was embarking on the type of nursing I had anticipated ever since the early days of my training; working in the community in people's own homes.

I had always felt that sometimes patients being treated in hospitals presented an artificial view of their overall mental and physical state. any cases needed the treatment only available in that environment, but equally in some cases I felt they would have responded more quickly and more completely in a home environment.

Many years in the future this has proved to be accepted by the medical profession.

I duly arrived at the District Nursing Headquarters on the appointed day and was introduced to an older senior nurse who would be my instructor and companion for a while until I took my exam, and then proved I was able to cope on my own. She was an attractive woman of about forty, I guessed, and told me she had been a district nurse for ten years. She was the sort of person I would have been comfortable with if I was a patient, giving the feeling of quiet efficiency. I decided that was how I would like to be.

Sandy first took me to the store to collect my uniform.

'You have three of these blue dresses, Chris....can I call you that?...six starched detachable collars and six starched aprons...then a winter coat, a blue cardigan, waterproof cape and the pillbox hat. You bring the collars and aprons here to be laundered and starched, but you are responsible for everything else. Any questions?'

'What sort of shoes, and do I wear my silver buckled belt?' (I was proud of that present from my parents after I had qualified.)

'Brown lace ups and black stockings, and of course wear your belt...and when you have passed the exam after a month's trial, you will be given the QIDN badge and striped chord so you can wear it round your neck under the collar. Now come along to the treatment room and we will sort a bag for you.'

After I had been allocated the aluminium navy canvas covered hinged bag and shown how to attach the linen removable internal cover, my mind was in a whirl. I hoped I would remember how to clip the lining in place and insert the dressing forceps and boilable syringe in the provided loops. Then I had to store enema funnel and equipment, bottles of saline for wound cleansing, bandages, mercurochrome for wounds and many other items. I began to realise how different this would be from nursing in a hospital, where all you had to do was go to a treatment room if you needed anything. Here you had to be sure you had everything with you at the patient's home or you did without, or had to cycle back to the rooms to collect what you had forgotten.

'What about dressings and sterilising the dressing forceps and syringes?'

'You boil the forceps, syringe and needles at the patient's home; I'll show you all that. Dressings; if a patient is due for frequent dressings, they get a metal biscuit tin from the grocer, you pack it for them and they sterilise in their oven, if they have one. Otherwise, we do it here in our autoclave. I don't suppose you know how to use one of those?'

I put Sandy right on that.

'Well, Chris that is enough for today. Come here at eight next Monday when we start and I will show you about checking your visiting list.' She indicated a complicated plan on the notice board. 'Hmm; looks as if you will be in the Tollington Park area; do you know it?'

I had cycled around some of the areas near home and had noticed several quite old blocks of tenement flats and rows and rows of terraced houses. I had also noticed a high proportion of immigrants walking the streets, and knew many West Indians and Greek Cypriots had settled there. I hoped I would be able to cope with the ethnic differences I knew I would be faced with. I had found so far, the only way was to treat everyone the same...as a patient needing my services... how could this be any different?

2/8

Monday arrived and dressed in my new uniform I caught the bus to the Headquarters, arriving at a quarter to eight. Sandy was there waiting for me and nodded with approval.

'Glad to see you are a good timekeeper. Now let's see who we have to visit.' She led me over to a pile of treatment notebooks and picked up one with *"Tollington Park Area"* stamped on the front.

'Now what you do is go and have a look on the notice board to see if any new patients are added for today.' She led the way and pointed to a list on the board. 'See if you can sort that while I have a look here in our notebook.'

I was not quite sure what I was looking for but dutifully scanned the list and saw 'Tollington Park' in red in a couple of places. I had a small notebook and pencil in my pocket so jotted the address, patient's name and treatment down then joined Sandy and showed her what I had done. She nodded and suggested I look through the treatment book as well. While I was doing that, I saw Sandy out of the corner of my eye checking the list on the notice board. I was a little annoyed but reasoned as it was my first day and she did not know me, it was fair enough.

Taking my list, the notebook, and a map of the whole area, Sandy gestured me over to a quiet corner. 'Now you need to plan your day.' For the next few minutes we studied the visits, including those from the notice board and I had to look up the addresses on the map. I was grateful Sandy was so patient with me as I had no idea where half the places were.

'You need also to put them in order of urgency. Your diabetic injections come first as a rule as they will be waiting to have their breakfast, and then I try to see the new ones in the morning. There's nothing worse than having to wait for your district nurse all day.' I was increasingly appreciative of Sandy and was grateful she was making such an effort on my behalf. I had hoped I would not be fobbed off with someone who might resent spending time with a new girl.

At last we were off and caught a bus to take us to the edge of our area: from there we would be walking. Sandy chatted as we travelled. 'I understand you have a bike, Chris? That will be quicker but it can get pretty chilly in the winter. You'd better invest in some "Witches Britches!" She laughed but I made a mental note to buy some thick long-legged pants the next time I was in "*Marks and Spencer's*."

The day went well, and I learned a few important details.

'I forgot to mention, make sure you check how you get into some of the homes.' Sandy showed me red notes by a few of the patients' names.'

'How d'you mean?'

'Sometimes the patient gives us a key to get in and it's left in the headquarters on a hook. You need to check before you set off, or you might have to go all the way back to get it.' She laughed, 'we all do it...just once.'

Then there was the approach to the patients themselves in their own home, which was quite different from treating them in hospital.

'Remember, you are a guest and there by invitation. Always respect that, especially as you will find some of the places a little different from what you are used to.'

I was increasingly amazed at the diversity of treatments we gave even in that one day. Our first patient was a diabetic who was not able to give herself the necessary insulin before she could have her breakfast. Normally a person's body manufactured the insulin which utilises sugars in the diet, but in a diabetic this does not happen so it has to be artificially introduced.

We visited several patients who needed dressing changes, and I was introduced to the technique. No pre sterilised instruments here; you had to do it yourself. The patient had a pan of water on the boil, with a cup and saucer placed in it. On our arrival, Sandy removed the instruments she would need form her bag and dropped them in the water making sure it kept to the boil and checking her watch. 'Five minutes boiling,' she explained as she folded a newspaper into an intricate receptacle which looked a little like a hat, and set in on the floor to receive the soiled dressing which she deftly removed. Placing the tin with the sterilised dressings supplied by the patient on a nearby table, she tipped the boiling water out of the pan, giving the contents a couple of minutes to cool. She then lifted the cup and saucer out, putting sterile dressings on one and cleansing lotion in the other. Finally, she picked up the forceps and completed cleaning and re-dressing the wound.

I asked how she managed the hot instruments; 'You get used to it after a while, but you can tip the instruments into the cleansing lotion first if you want, to cool.' She laughed, 'My fingers are so insulated by now I can handle hot plates and utensils much to the distress of others I might hand them to.'

Next we called in to an elderly couple, where sadly the old lady was dying of cancer. I called to mind my earlier conviction that some cases were better nursed at home, and this was one of them. The daughter was staying in the small home, sleeping on a mattress on the lounge floor and managing very well, with a little advice from the district nurses. Our visit was a daily one to wash the old lady and attend to anything else needed.

'I want me mum to die at 'ome. S'the best I can do after all she done for us kids. There was ten of us, it's just me brother and me here now.'

That thought kept coming back to me as for the rest of the week I trotted around after Sandy, gradually being give more to do, and learned about the area where I would be working. Some houses we visited had been large family homes in Victorian times, now divided into apartment and bedsitting rooms, or 'bedsits'. These consisted of a single room which doubled as bedroom and sitting room, often with a corner screened off as a kitchen which might contain a cooker and sink if you were lucky, but more likely a gas ring and jug and bowl. Toilets were shared and possibly a general bathroom with gas geyser to heat the water and a slot meter to give a few inches of tepid water for a bath. Occasionally there might be a house phone in the entrance hall, but more likely you had to look for a public call box that worked. Most of them did, too, as vandalism was not a big issue as you never knew when a public phone would be needed.

Many of these houses were occupied by immigrants, and they were overfilled with their relatives. I wondered how they ever survived, packed two and three families to a bedsit. Treating people in the tenement flats also had its problems as basic hygiene was difficult and sometimes abandoned altogether.

I realised as the week progressed I had a lot to learn.

2/9

For another week Sandy accompanied me, allowing me to sort my visits and give all the treatment. At the end she congratulated me.

'You have a nice way with people, you know. You never talk down to them as some young people do. I am sure you will manage well, providing you can find your way around alright.' She laughed and I grinned sheepishly, as I still had trouble locating some of the houses. 'I think you are ready for your exam.'

My heart flipped a little, but I reasoned Sandy would not suggest it if she thought I was not ready. In fact it was not difficult; mainly covering things I had already done with Sandy, plus a Fist Aid test. I had taken a Red Cross course while I was working at the outpatients' department, as it was a requirement, so that was no problem.

After a month, I was on my own.

I had given my trusty Moulton bike a thorough overhaul. The last thing I wanted was a problem with it halfway round my visits. It was ideal for my new work, as the nursing bag fitted on the back carrier, and the side pannier I had used on holiday was useful for any equipment I needed in addition. Sometimes I had to pack in dressings if the patient could not sterilise them and there were extra bottles of wound cleansing liquid to carry.

At first I was a little anxious but I had got to know a few regular patients by then and it was warming to be greeted as an anticipated visitor. I had heard of the sociability of Londoners but that did not seem to apply to my area. Sometimes the district nurse would be the only person seen that day. In cases like that, I tried to find time to stop for a cup of tea and a chat, but it was not always possible, and accepting refreshment was always a difficult situation. The basic hygiene so often was just that; very basic. Several of the houses had no running water, just a communal tap, and water had to be collected from a standpipe nearby for everything, so its use was often minimal.

Nursing people in their own homes was a revelation. Coping with the difficult sanitary arrangements, people made the best of the situation as everyone was in the same boat. The bugs and bacteria had not learned to be resistant; children played in the mud and did not get ill; boiling instruments and baking dressings seemed to sterilize sufficiently, and any bugs in the home belonged there where the residents had developed their own resistance.

It was very rare for wounds to become infected.

Most of the people were not well off and sometimes in the colder weather stayed huddled in bed as the cold autumn weather arrived and I was glad of my purchase from *"Marks and Spencer's."* With my thick black stockings and warm pants, I managed to ward off the worst of the cold air as I cycled from patient to patient.

One day I had to give an injection to an old lady I had not visited before. The door was unlocked so I pushed it open, calling out 'District Nurse!' and followed the muffled reply into a darkened room. There were heavy curtains at the window to keep in what little heat there was, and I could just see the tousled bed in the corner where my patient was apparently huddled to keep warm.

I prepared the syringe by boiling it, and when it was cool, drew up the Vitamin B12 due for my patient. I then called over to the bed, 'Mrs Popolous, just stick your leg out of the bed, no need to come out in the cold.' A leg was duly extended and I gave the injection, but as I turned round to pack my things away, two more heads appeared from the mound of bedclothes.

For a moment I stood transfixed, and only hoped I had given it to the right patient!

Treating people in the tenement flats I discovered also had its problems as basic hygiene was difficult and sometimes abandoned altogether. One recurring problem was leg ulcers in the elderly. It was virtually impossible to keep them clean and sterile. These often appeared when a scratch would not heal due to poor circulation in the lower limbs, and then infection crept in.

I was asked one day to call and see a lady who had ulcers on both legs. She was in one of the older blocks of tenement flats and I decided not to risk the lift, walking up the two flights of stairs instead. All the front doors faced on to an open corridor where you could look down to the ground where teenagers collected in groups, smoking and calling to each other. I found the door to the flat with difficulty as some of the numbers had been removed and knocked several times. No answer. I pushed the door, which opened and called the lady's name, nearly gagging at the strong smell of urine which wafted from the rooms beyond.

'In here, deary; oo is it?'

'Queen's district nurse.'

The patient was enormous, half sitting, half lying in a filthy chair, legs propped on a wooden box.

'Sorry, can't get up. It's me legs, ye see. An' 'ow is the dear Lady, then?'

I had become used by then to people asking after our Queen Elizabeth's health and had to disillusion patients, by explaining I had not just come hotfoot from Buckingham Palace. It had amused me at first until I realised many Londoners really believed their Queen called on our services and were secretly proud to be at one with royalty.

I looked with horror at the swollen, weeping legs. Ulcers encircled each leg almost from knee to ankle, with dirty dressings draped around. There was a strong smell of urine, and I realised part of the moisture was from external contamination.

'I can't get down ye see; I catches me legs.'

I did the best I could and hoped I had made things a little more comfortable, but it was a little like trying to treat a gaping wound with a sticking plaster. I knew next day the situation would be as bad and we nurses would be calling for years, never seeing any improvement. Mrs Betts enjoyed the visits, and I was able to spend a little time chatting but I drew the line at a cup of tea on this occasion.

As Sandy had advised me, I was very careful to check the means of getting into a patient's home before I set off on my rounds. I did forget a key...just once. A sound lesson which I regretted all the way back to the rooms to collect it.

Other instructions were sometimes a little vague. *"Key through letter box",* had me wondering, but I assumed it was hanging inside on a string for this particular new patient. I was right; what the instructions failed to say was that there was a large dog also in the house. Each time I opened the letterbox flap and put my hand through, the dog started to bark, and I could feel his hot breath on my hand. After several attempts I was becoming frustrated and angry; I had a lot of visits to do. I do not normally swear but remembering some of Sir Spaggs' language I suddenly shouted through the open letter box, giving the dog some of the surgeon's best, ending by shouting, *'Oh b....ger off you stupid dog!'* He yelped and shot off under the patient's bed, refusing to move until I left.

After that we understood each other on my next visits.

2/10

As the weeks passed, I realised much of my work was social, though there were of course social workers, but they were thin on the ground. We nurses, who visited frequently, often had a pulse on the home environment. Sometimes it was difficult not to become too involved.

It was nearing Christmas of my first year as a district nurse and I had a young single parent family in my care. Josie had cancer and it was unlikely she would see another year. It had started in her breast, but she was one of the unlucky ones, and it had been quite aggressive, moving through her body. Treatment had only slowed the inevitable outcome.

Josie was always cheerful and cared for her six-year-old daughter Suzie, and four-year old son Paul with all the little energy she had. Somehow the young woman remained pretty, despite her loss of weight, and I wondered how her husband could have left her with a young family. She told me when she had been diagnosed with cancer he could not cope and had left with her best friend.

'You know Chris; the old story. I got pregnant with Suzie and Jerry did the 'right thing' by marrying me. It was alright at first, I think he did love me in his way, but then when Paul came along it was too much for him. Then I got this cancer and that was that.' There was no self-pity and I mentally cursed the selfishness of some men.

The three of them lived in a tiny bedsit right at the top of a house, with the kitchen just on the landing. It was always spotless, but as the festive season approached Suzie became more and more withdrawn. Finally, I tackled her, and she admitted she did not know how to give her children a special Christmas, as she knew it may be her last.

'The trouble is, Chris, I just have not the energy to shop and cook the dinner, or get presents, even if I had the money.'

I thought for a while and then had an idea. 'Just leave it with me.'

Next club day I told the young people about my problem. 'That's OK Mrs Chris' several exclaimed; 'We'll sort it'. And they did. A whip-round produced a few cuddly toys, some games and a small train set which the youngsters said they had spare. Again, my admiration grew for these young people who had little themselves. Ken and I bought a few sweets; the social department had offered money to buy a chicken and vegetables and I had a spare pudding as I usually made mine. We were due to have an evening meal with Ken's parents, so it fitted in well.

On Christmas Day several of us went late in the morning and cooked the Christmas lunch. It was a jolly time and it was wonderful to see the children's faces as they unwrapped their presents, and then we left the young family as they settled to their meal.

I had several days leave due, so it was a week before I called to see Suzie again. I was surprised she had not been on my visiting list, but assumed someone else had been visiting in my absence. I called in anyway, but as I walked up the stairs it was strangely silent.

'They've gone.' A woman poked her head out of the door on a lower floor as she heard my footsteps, taking round the cigarette in her mouth. 'Noisy little brats and that mother a lazy cow; spent most of 'er time in bed, didn't she?'

I tried to curb my irritation with the woman, as she blew smoke out of the corner of her mouth.

'Where have they gone?'

'She collapsed and she went off to hospital, didn't she? Kids've gone into care.'

I felt my eyes prickle as I quickly let myself out of the house. I knew I should not get involved, but how could you give care without compassion? I had to learn the hard way the optimum balance of care and disassociation, though I could not avoid developing affection for some of the patients.

One such was old Mrs Pettigrew. At 90 she still had an acute interest in anything I would care to talk about. Blind and a survivor of bowel cancer, she was unable to care for the colostomy which had been necessary to save her life. This unpleasant artificial bowel opening in the lower abdomen had to have a bag attached and changed on a daily basis; a totally impossible activity for the old lady. The problem was she sometimes tried to change it, or on occasion it leaked, so, often there was an unpleasant mess to clear up and sometimes her hands showed the evidence. She had indoor plumbing and an old stone sink, although her toilet was outside and she managed well in her three-roomed downstairs flat and knew where everything was. So I had to make sure I did not move anything from its accustomed place.

Often I tried to allow a longer visit than the usual fifteen minutes as I needed tact to make the old, sensitive lady comfortable. So we chatted while I gave treatment while she told me of her life as a teacher in Canada.

'You know Sister Chris, life was pretty rough then, bit like the Wild West. The children often had to ride miles to attend school, and we had a paddock for the horses during the day.'

'What about winter?'

'Ah well, it was sledges then, you see. We had this old wood stove in the centre of the room and used to sit round it for lessons.'

I wondered how Mrs Pettigrew had ended in a small flat in London, and one day she told me.

'My Charlie was a logger: a lovely man and the love of my life.' She grew pensive as I gently continued with her treatment. 'Then there was the accident and my world fell apart; my father wanted me back home as my mother was ill, so I came.' She turned her blind eyes to me and I saw a small tear run down her cheek. 'I carried on teaching here in London after she died and looked after dad.' She gripped my arm. 'Make sure you value your husband, Sister Chris; you don't know how long you'll have,'

One day when I arrived, she was excited.

'Guess what, Sister Chris,' she exclaimed as I walked in the door, 'the local social workers think I need a holiday and I am off next week to a rest home in Brighton for a week. I haven't a thing to wear!'

I laughed and suggested we have a look after the treatment was finished. She guided me to her tidy bedroom and flung open the door of a large wardrobe. It was filled with good quality clothes, and I spent a little time describing them to her and finally Mrs Pettigrew made the choice, but was a little distressed that they smelled strongly of mothballs. I promised to wash and iron them for her and we spent an exciting week planning her first holiday in years.

While she was away I missed my regular visits and was pleased when Betty Pettigrew returned, although I knew part of the plan was to try and introduce the idea of a rest home on a permanent basis.

The old lady was quiet while I attended to her needs, and as we sat down for a cup of tea, I asked her how she had enjoyed herself.

'Well, dear, it was very nice, but I prefer my own home.' She smiled a little to herself. 'Mind you it had its moments; there was a lovely man there that was very friendly; he asked me to marry him.'

I looked at the old lady in surprise. 'Well, and did you accept?'

'Oh no, dear, he was far too young. He was only 75!'

For the rest of the day this returned to give me great amusement, and I was secretly relieved I would not be losing one of my favourite patients just yet.

I tried not to have favourites, but I found the old man who lived in the flat above Mrs Pettigrew difficult and taciturn. I only had to visit him on one occasion, and he would not let me into the bedroom. I had a small dressing to do and so agreed to stay in the kitchen.

Some months afterwards, I learned he had been admitted into an old people's home and a social worker arrived to sort out his belongings. I was attending to Betty Pettigrew when the social worker whom I knew, came rushing downstairs.

'Quick, Chris come upstairs; I need your help!'

Bemused I followed her into the bedroom. There was money everywhere; spilling from drawers; sticking out of a vase and even peeping from under the mattress.

'What on earth…?'

'He had social security extra payments as we thought he needed the money; apparently he did not!"

We counted over 400 pounds, a small fortune in those days. I could not help but wonder at a system which had apparently not checked on a person's needs. We bundled up the notes and the social worker went off in her little car and I continued with my rounds on my bicycle. I did not envy her driving around London, except in the winter and when it was raining.

2/11

I had settled quite happily in my district nursing and enjoyed the diversity of treatment given in patients' homes, but in the back of my mind I knew I would not want to live in London for the rest of my working life. I had always been a country girl at heart, growing up mostly with the rural background of 'Shakespeare Country,' in Warwickshire; the heart of England. I had attended village schools and even my grammar school was set in Shottery, the lovely rural village where Shakespeare's wife, Anne Hathaway had lived.

I missed the countryside, although we did continue our cycling Youth Hostel holidays and even had another trip overseas; this time to Andalucía in Spain. Again, we went with a Youth Hostel Holiday trip, with a guide. It was in October and despite pre-booking the hostels, most of them had decided to close, presumably not wanting to bother for a group of ten or so. The guide had contingency funds and we ended up in small *"pensions"* or local small hotels instead. This of course was an advantage for Ken and me, as we were able to share a room, instead of being in separate dormitories.

The facilities were not luxurious, but enabled us to meet local people. The rooms of one, in Seville, faced directly onto a courtyard and there was just a heavy double door opening onto it and no windows, so we had to suffer hot nights or be visible to anyone in the courtyard. On the first night I noticed a small wooden shutter high on the back wall.

'Look, Ken; maybe that's a window; can you try to open it?'

With a little pulling he did, only to find himself looking straight into the kitchen and the face of someone working there, which was rather embarrassing as they would have heard everything we had said or done.

I loved the Spanish villages and towns with their whitewashed walls and red tiled roofs, delighting in the

Alhambra and the Generalife Palaces in Granada, with their many fountains and water features, so different from anything in England. Ken had been reading about the architecture and style.

'You know much of this was built by the Moors who believed nothing should be perfect, so apparently the people who did the tiling were told to make a few mistakes in the design. It says here you can find them if you look hard.' Try as we might, neither of us could discover any mistakes.

The Spanish food was quite different too, with several courses, often with the meat served separately, and it was the custom to eat late at night. We were used to our evening meal about seven, but in Spain we often did not sit down until ten for the first course, which was usually a salad of thinly sliced tomatoes, onion and garlic, with an olive oil dressing. Then came fried potatoes then the meat. Sometimes we were offered a steaming bowl of soup, which had a whole raw egg broken into it, or if it was fish, the whole prawns, whiskers and all, staring at us with their shoe-button eyes.

It was fun also to visit the markets, which were always colourful and noisy, reminding me a little of Petticoat Lane in London, with punters trying to sell their wares. As we wandered around, Ken took a fancy to a large shallow brass dish hanging in one stall. We thought it was a dish used to cook the delicious Spanish Paella, a speciality of saffron rice, fish and chicken which we had all enjoyed.

'Look, Chris: wouldn't that look good hung on the wall?'

'How on earth will you carry it?'

'On the back of my backpack.'

Despite my efforts to dissuade him Ken was uncharacteristically stubborn and bought the thing, although he paid what was asked without bargaining, which I would have done.

As I had expected, it caused some adverse comment as we progressed down the train corridors on the next part of our trip and I think later he may have regretted his purchase.

We finished our holiday in Barcelona and we decided to try to buy some sweet Malaga wine to take home. It was not easy to locate, but we were directed to an area away from popular streets where there were large warehouses and groups of men sitting around playing cards. I felt rather nervous, but eventually we did manage to buy a bottle and I was glad to escape to The Ramblas area and more people.

This went into Ken's backpack, which proved not to be such a good idea.

As we were sitting in the train on our way home, I noticed a small puddle seeping from Ken's rucksack on the floor. We discovered the brass dish had been banging on the bottle and cracked it. Poor Ken had sticky clothes, and we had to throw the cherished bottle away.

My comment, 'Just as well we are on the way home,' was not received enthusiastically.

It was an enjoyable time but when we returned home we began to think what we would like to do in the future. I had been district nursing for about five years and Ken was at a time in his advertising work where he was regarded as an 'old man' in a young man's profession. He had done wonderfully well, working from office boy to junior executive but he knew he had climbed as far up the ladder as he could. The new recruits were mostly ex-university, and more socially inclined than my rather reticent husband. Part of his responsibility was to take clients out to lunch and win their interest, and he was not really a social animal, never having had the training or opportunity.

'I don't know how long they will keep me on, Chris.'
'So what do you want to do, then?'
'I'd like to have a business of our own.'
'Like what?'

'Maybe a guest house somewhere?'

The vision of all that housework did not appeal to me at all, although I loved to cook, so I said: 'Not unless it was on Sark', thinking that possibility was safely remote. We had visited that tiny feudal Island again several times, as well as on our honeymoon, and each time we had both fallen more deeply under its magic spell.

To my surprise Ken did not laugh, but just said; 'Now there's a thought.'

For a while we continued with our work, but when the next holiday was discussed we both agreed to return to Sark, with an intention of discovering what sort of properties might be for sale, and at what price.

The outcome was totally unexpected and within a year we had bought a property on Sark, moved there, and opened a guest house. There we stayed for seven years, and then took off to visit New Zealand with young son Roy who had been born in 1968, for two years until 1974. On our return, having decided to emigrate, we were back in London for a few months. I had discovered if I wanted to be a district nurse in New Zealand I would need some midwifery qualification, although it was not necessary to be a fully qualified midwife.

In those days in the United Kingdom, the midwifery training was split it two parts. For the first six months students worked in a hospital environment, witnessing births then delivering a specified number of babies. You were then qualified to work as a hospital midwife, but to be fully qualified it was necessary to spend another six months in the community with a district midwife.

I would only need 'part one' as it was called, so approached St Mary's wing at the Whittington hospital, where I had worked in the outpatients' department before.

The only problem was where we would live, but Ken's mother kindly suggested we move in with her in Finchley for the duration. His father had died, and I think Elsie was rather lonely, although she had relatives over the road, and lived for her Methodist church. It was a bonus for her to have her only grandchild to spoil, and Roy would be able to attend the local school. Another bonus was his wakening interest in learning to play his Nana's piano, and we were happy to pay for lessons, which he was to keep up for many years.

Ken managed to get a job with the local parks gardeners and soon oversaw several of them.

The only problem was the distance between Finchley and Holloway, which was about six miles. 'I'll buy a motorbike,' I announced to a sceptical Ken and Elsie. 'Just a small 50cc should be enough to ferry me, and I can put an extra seat on the back for Roy.'

So that is what I did.

I bought us both helmets and I wrapped myself into a set of black 'leathers' in case I came off in the road. Roy and I had some fun when I was not on duty driving around the area.

When I was on my way to the hospital the bike was light enough for me to hop off if I was stopped by a long queue of cars at a red light. I would just push it up the pavement to the head of the stationary cars, probably to the displeasure of the other drivers.

2/12

On the first day of my midwifery training, we were collected into the classroom by the tutor. I realised I was considerably older than many of the students, as most were immigrants, qualified in their own country but needing to have six months' nursing experience before being admitted onto the English Nursing Register.

The Midwifery tutor asked us to talk a little about our most recent nursing experience, and when it came to my turn, I was a little hesitant, as I realised I was much more experienced than any of the others.

'Er, well I was a matron of a small medical and post operative hospital in Auckland, New Zealand.'

The sister raised her eyebrows, and I had a feeling she was not too pleased with my answer as she said sharply.

'You are just a junior again and you are here under instruction. I hope you can cope with that, nurse.'

To which I replied meekly, 'I am here to learn, sister.'

Learn I did, as my age and experience ensured I obtained more than the younger students. Often there would be two of us on duty on a ward, but usually the other nurse would not take the responsibility to be in charge, which did not worry me. I did not push myself, but usually the younger nurses refused to make any decisions, and several of them could hardly speak English anyway.

There were two anti-natal wards and two post-natal wards.

On the anti-natal ward the patients were awaiting delivery with problems which required careful monitoring. Pre-eclampsia, when a pregnant woman's blood pressure became too high, and with oedema...swelling of tissues, and the presence of albumin in the urine, it could mean a premature birth, loss of the baby or even death of the young mother. It was a condition I was all too familiar with, as this had happened at the birth of my son Roy, and he was born prematurely while I was quite ill. I sympathised with these young women who had to be kept calm and quiet, and especially as they were on a bland low salt diet, to try to reduce the excessive fluid in their tissues, a side effect of a too high blood pressure.

Other conditions requiring hospitalisation included 'placenta previa' when there might be a danger of severe bleeding during delivery. In this condition, the placenta...afterbirth... is situated over or partially over the birth channel and could rupture during the birth causing severe bleeding.

There were also women with expected multiple births as it was felt it was safer in a hospital environment.

The post-natal ward was more enjoyable as usually the babies stayed with their mothers unless they needed to be in an incubator in the special baby nursery. Here we had to help the young mothers with feeding and other techniques, which I had experienced first-hand, but most of the young trainee nurses did not have that advantage. I had problems with my young premature son and sympathised with those who had a baby who would not stop crying, and I was able to pass on a few tips.

Besides lectures...bringing back memories of my student days...we had to observe a certain number of deliveries before we were allowed to be involved ourselves under supervision. We would have a call such as, *"Delivery in theatre one,"* and off we would race to the appropriate location arriving out of breath, quickly to tie on waterproof aprons, masks, and hair coverings. The theatre would often be very hot and on one occasion I began to feel a little faint after the rush from my ward. Looking at the red sweating face of the young woman on the delivery table I suggested turning the fan on for her, which also saved me.

When I had seen enough babies born, I was delighted to be able to attend to the twenty or so deliveries I needed to perform, to be able to take the examination at the end of six months. I had made my first delivery several years ago on Sark, in an emergency and now I realised how wrong everything might have gone. I had been shown a few films about emergency births in my district nursing training, and had bought a book, which had been a great help in Sark. I now realised the chord could have strangled the baby, or there have been post-partum problems. Now I learned in detail the miraculous event of a birth.

As soon as the baby was ready to be born, and the crown of its head was visible, careful control of the mother's wish to bear down was important, to avoid a tear of her tissues. Then the head was delivered, and I always felt it was a miracle first to see the funny red-faced baby's head appearing, often shooting out a mouthful of amniotic fluid from its mouth. We were taught always to see if the chord had wound round the baby's neck while in the birth canal. If not slipped back over the baby's head, possibly the baby would strangle during delivery. One of mine proved how important that was, as there were three loops round the baby's neck as the chord must have been exceptionally long.

Sometimes there were complications, like a breech delivery, when the baby presented legs and bottom first. I only had one in my deliveries, and I was exhausted but elated by the time the baby was born. At a time like that, or if the baby was large, we had to perform an episiotomy, a cut to widen the birth canal, or the tissue might tear, causing very unpleasant side effects to the mother.

In those days, husbands were not allowed in the delivery ward as a general rule, but sometime a member of the family had to act as interpreter. Many of the families in that area were immigrants from Cyprus and I had worked among them as a district nurse, enjoying their hospitality and the delicious Turkish coffee they made. The problem was, the women were not encouraged to learn English by the husbands, so it was impossible to have their cooperation during the delivery. The situation sometimes arose for a schoolboy to be used as interpreter, which was far from ideal.

I enjoyed my short time as a student midwife but did not think I would like to have acted as a district midwife as I really enjoyed the variety in general district nursing. I passed the examination well and earned a grudging congratulation from the sister tutor. I am not sure what her problem was, but I was glad to leave the training school.

I decided to have a couple of weeks with my parents in Yorkshire to recover from the intensive six months, taking Roy with me so his other grandparents could enjoy their only grandchild.

Ken decided to stay in London with his work.

We caught the train to the north and Roy had another session of being spoiled, this time by my parents, but I was very sad to see my father's Parkinson's disease had deteriorated. He was still able to play a little golf and drove his precious old Daimler...his pride and joy...around the district, but I could see he was looking older. My lovely stepmother was sad we had decided to go to New Zealand, but as she said, 'Chrissie, you must lead your own life.' She asked me about Ken, knowing I was not very happy in my marriage.

'The trouble is, I was so young and naive when we married and Ken was the man he was going to be. We just seem to be on parallel lines now, but we have Roy to think of.'

'Do you think running off the New Zealand will help?'

'A new life; maybe things will be different.'

'Well they weren't in Sark, were they?'

I remembered again all our cherished dreams when we had first arrived in that little Island. How hard we had worked and how successful our guest house and eventual smallholding had been. Then I had become pregnant, and things had started to go wrong.

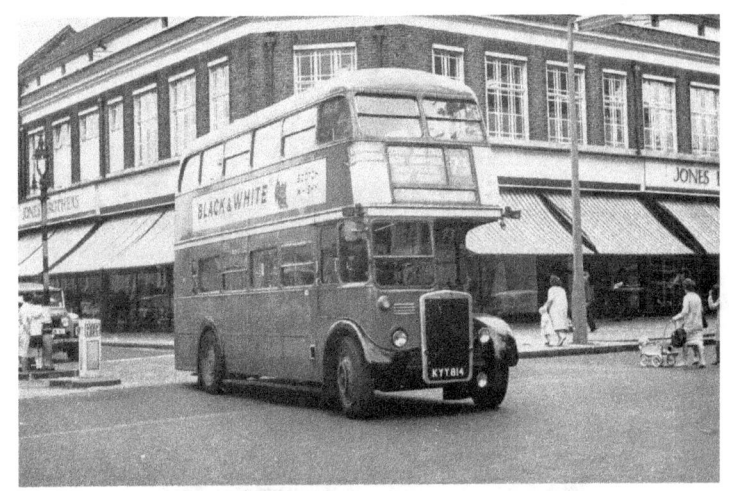

London Bus circa 1960

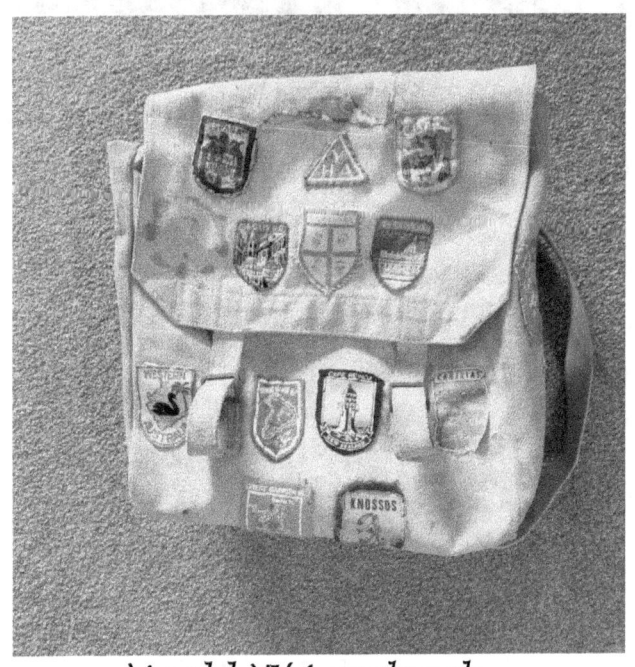

My old YHA rucksack

PART 3
SARK
1966-1972 and 1984-2009

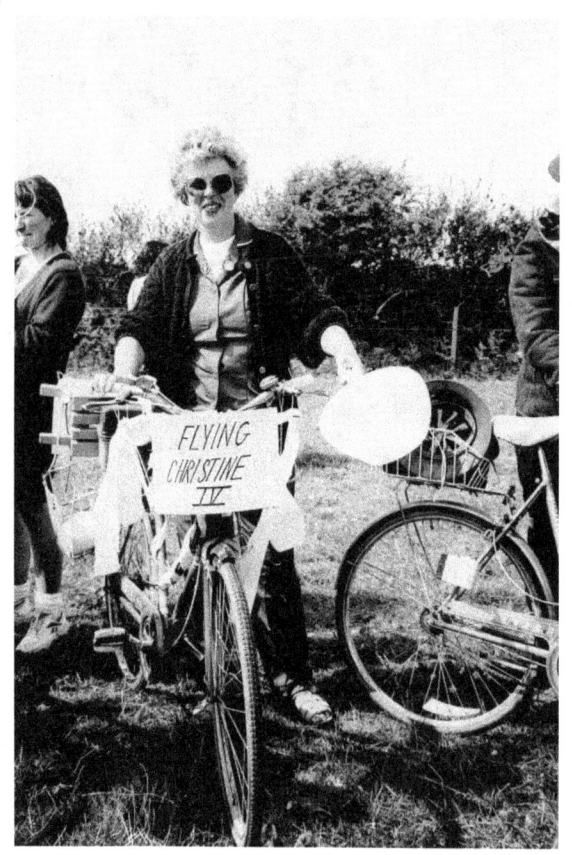

*District Nursing Sark style
(The St John Ambulance launch
was called "Flying Christine 3")*

3/1

Our trip to Sark in 1965 was mainly designed to look at the sort of properties which came onto the market, to assess the price and if we would ever be able to afford to move there one day.

It did not happen that way.

We knew the ownership of houses was unique and dated way back four hundred years. At that time the Island was a haunt of pirates but good Queen Elizabeth the First realised the Channel Islands' proximity to France was advantageous. She decided it was time to populate Sark with forty landowners, or *'Tenants,'* controlled by a *'Seigneur'*, or governor. She chose one Helier de Carteret from the neighbouring Island of Jersey, and Sark was split into forty *'Tenements,'* each having some good land and some cliff or *'cotile'*

We discovered Sark was still divided into those original forty Tenements, and it was against Sark law for the owners to sub-divide and sell off a piece, but leases could be negotiated. Some landowners just leased off the land, and houses were built on that land. The only problem with that was when a land lease expired the house may have to be moved. In other cases, the whole property was on a rental, either annually or for a lump sum for a specified number of years.

Although theoretically all the land had been divided it appeared some small pockets of freehold had escaped. Such a one was 'Le Clos Des Camps,' which had a freehold two-acre piece of land and a wooden bungalow built by the 'Colt' company in 1946. We had heard of this type of building, which was prefabricated in sections and finished with cedar shingles on external walls and roof. Not an inexpensive form of building, but on an island where everything had to be ferried from the UK to Guernsey and then to Sark, it was a much more sensible plan than building all from scratch.

It was this property we finally bought, just a few days before we were due to depart back to London at the end of our holiday in 1965.

As the holiday progressed, we had found our time mostly taken with searching for properties on the market, and even several which were not, as several had been pointed out to us as possibilities. The more we looked the keener we were to find somewhere; the magic of the island had bewitched us. It was an Arcadian May, with hot sun tempered by refreshing breezes, and the whole Island ablaze with wildflowers.

We had been told 'Le Clos des Camps' was for sale but we had rejected it as it seemed too small when we peeped into the garden in passing. A huge rough lawn in front dominated the bungalow which was set back at its edge. There was a small, covered porch at the front over the main door and a lean-to sunroom to the right, but there were only three windows showing and Ken remarked;

'If those windows are the only bedrooms, it won't be big enough.'

We had decided by then we would have to take paying guests and I had accepted the inevitable most likely means of income, at least at the beginning, although I had hopes of nursing, too.

We visited a lovely building called 'The Barracks' but the lease was too much for our purse, and even an old farmhouse nearby, but then discovered a stream ran through the kitchen. In desperation, with only a few days left of our holiday, we agreed to have a look at 'Le Clos des Camps.'

Access to the lawn was through a small gate set between two banks topped with veronica hedges, at that time of year full of lovely deep purple flowers. Two big flower beds either side of the lawn were mostly planted with what I had learned were lupine trees, a wild species of the garden vari-coloured plants. These were large bushes with the distinctive flower in shades of white and yellow and I had been told they thrived in the salty air near the sea. The property was open to the view of the islands of Guernsey and Herm across the sea with just a few hydrangea bushes near the house.

As we approached, the owners, Mr and Mrs Morris opened the door in the front porch and walked down to meet us. Having shaken hands and admired the view, we were escorted into the bungalow. To our surprise the place was much bigger than we had realised with four bedrooms, a largish lounge, bathroom with toilet, long kitchen, large storeroom and pantry and a sunroom which ran the whole length of one side.

'I understand you used to run this as a guest house?' I enquired of Mrs Morris. She appeared the typical 'landlady' with rosy cheeks and a ready smile.

'Yes, my dear; but it got too much for my hubby who has a bit of a heart, you know.'

I tried not to smile and knew what she meant. She continued, 'I understand that is what you want to do?'

I hesitated a little, as I still was not sure about my feelings regarding housework but assumed this place would not be too difficult to look after, as it was only one floor. I still had hopes of acting as a district nurse, so I asked if there was a nursing service already on Sark.

'Not as such. We just have the one doctor and in the past his wife did a bit. Then there was nurse Donovan, who was a retired district nurse, and now Mrs Pratt who is also retired does as much as she can. People must go over to Guernsey, you know.'

At that stage I did not want to say anything more, but it all sounded promising.

After a cup of tea and a wander round the two large fields which were part of the property, Ken and I thoughtfully returned to the old farmhouse 'La Ville Farm' where we were staying. Mr and Mrs French had become friends during the several times we had visited, and so we told them about 'Le Clos des Camps' and our thoughts. They were an interesting couple; between them they had lived in France, Guernsey and Jersey, and their conversation was peppered with patois and French.

'*Alors,* Chris, it is hard work *tu sais.* You are never really off the duty when you have guests in: but you are used to people and you are both young, *n'est pas?*'

That night Ken and I talked into the night, discussing pros and cons. By morning we had decided to make an offer.

'But will your dad transfer his loan, Ken?'

'I think he will. I had a little chat with him before we left.'

'You mean you had thought we might find somewhere? You didn't say anything to me.'

'I didn't want to raise your hopes.'

'That's not the point. I thought we were supposed to share everything?' I said nothing more but was secretly rather hurt. I sometime felt Ken was still behaving as a bachelor, which he had been for so many years before we were married. I would just have to be patient and hope he would eventually change.

As soon as we had finished the huge breakfast of bacon, eggs, tomatoes, and crispy fried bread, followed by mounds of toast and home-made marmalade, we telephoned Mr and Mrs Morris and asked if we could call in again to see them.

For a while we negotiated, then finally came to an agreement to buy the freehold for seven thousand pounds. Dazed we returned to the Farmhouse and announced to the French's.

'We have an agreement to buy 'Le Clos des Camps.'

The old couple hugged us and admitted they had not thought we were serious. 'You know *beaucoup* people say they want to live here, but seldom follow it through, *tu sais'*

Ken and I went for a walk and discussed our plans.

'The only problem is we need to sell Tabley Rd, persuade Dad to transfer the loan and move within six months, as Sark law decrees.'

'And we must pay the *'thresieme'.'* I reminded Ken. This was a sort of Island tax purchasers of a freehold had to add to the purchase price...a thirteenth part of the agreed price.

We returned to London two days later, a little stunned at what we had done, but determined to make a go of this new adventure.

3/2

On our return to London, Ken and I immediately went to see his father. Dear man, there was no hesitation in agreeing to transfer his loan. I always felt he would have liked Ken to follow in his footsteps in the building business, and I am sure he would have done well as he was very handy with tools. Elsie, on the other hand had wanted him to aim higher, as she saw it, and encouraged his moving into the 'white collar' working world. Be that as it may, Ken and his father did not always see eye to eye but I think he was secretly pleased his only son was showing some enterprise in launching out in his own business. Elsie was not happy with our proposed plan, and I think always blamed me for persuading Ken to abandon his career. In fact, it was mainly Ken's instigation as he knew his advertising days were numbered, and it showed courage to take on this challenge. Having worked his way up to junior management, he was one of the older staff in a young man's world. Ken did not give in his notice immediately, as it was an advantage to stay on until the end of the financial year to benefit from a tax refund, so he planned to travel to Sark to see me settled, then return and stay with his parents until Easter.

Our next responsibility was to sell our house, and so we approached the sales offices with a little anxiety. Inevitably, England was suffering from a slight depression, and we needed to get as much as possible to cover the purchase of Clos des Camps, the Sark tax and moving expenses as well. For several months we showed people round our first home together and eventually we found a buyer, but had to reduce the price as time was running out. We had a shortfall of about one thousand pounds.

Ken's father helped us out again there, adding our debt to what we already owed him, without asking for interest payments.

My supervisors were not too pleased when I told them I would be leaving, but after a while the Charge Sister became interested in my plans.

'You say there is not a district nurse on the Island, Christine?'

'Well it is only one and a half miles wide and three long with a population of five hundred you know.'

'But how do people manage for medical needs?'

'There is one doctor and up to now there has usually been a retired nurse to help him. Otherwise, they have to go to Guernsey, the nearest island. St John has a sort of motorboat ambulance, the *Flying Christine*'

'Surely the National Health Service could send a nurse over?'

'Ah well that's the problem. No UK National services on Sark. No health or unemployment, social services and so on.'

'How strange; so how do people manage?'

I shrugged as I was not quite sure how the system worked, yet. I did know we had been advised to take out private medical insurance and arrange to pay our social security contributions as 'overseas residents.' For all our working lives we had contributed to the British government's system of the National Health Service, which provided free medical treatment, unemployment benefit, social services, and a pension in old age. Now we would have none of these while we were living on Sark. Paying as overseas residents with a smaller contribution, would ensure at least a pension when we reached the ages of sixty for me and sixty-five for Ken. At twenty-six it seemed a long time in the future, but as Ken explained;

'We don't know what lies ahead.'

Eventually the Charge Sister became interested in my plan to try to start a private district nursing service and advised me to contact the Royal College of Nursing, which controlled the activities of registered nurses in the United Kingdom.

'You will need to know what your fees should be, and I expect they may let you use the QIDN badge, and I am sure they will let you have a couple of uniforms and a nursing bag. You may need to buy your own instruments, though. I'll give you the address where you can get some.' She directed me to Charring Cross Road where there were several medical instrument suppliers.

Taking a break from packing, I happily found my way on the underground to the heart of London. Among the bustle of this big city, where I felt perfectly at home, I felt a strange detachment. I realised within a few months all this would be replaced by a rural cottage on a remote island. Gone would be the commuters sitting staring into space as the train rattled from station to station. The busy people-choked streets would give way to country lanes and the noisy vehicles would be replaced by the clip clop of horses' hooves.

I could not wait.

I wrote to the RCN, but it had repercussions, as I discovered some time after we moved to Sark.

In the meantime there was a lot to do. We had arranged to buy some furniture from Mr and Mrs Morris, but we would need cutlery and crockery, bed linen, pillows, pans and much more. We spent all our spare time visiting sales and suppliers and were fortunate the big store of Gamages in Holborn near where Ken worked, had a sale of sheets and pillowcases. It was only later I discovered the beautifully crisp and white linen had to be ironed while damp, to keep the crispness. There would be no laundry to help in Sark.

Crockery was a problem, as matching replacements would be difficult to obtain in the Channel Isles where supplies were much less than in London, but Ken hit on the idea of purchasing Melamine. This looked like china but was unbreakable, and the style we chose was prettily patterned with Wedgewood blue and white main theme. It was to serve us well, but I was always a little conscious it really was a sort of plastic. Blue and white damask-like tablecloths and serviettes in easy care Terylene kept the colour theme. We had plans to decorate the sunroom at the side of our new home, in matching colours and use it as the dining room.

Finally, we had to think of our proposed income from paying guests. Here Ken's experience came in handy. Advertisements were placed in the 'Lady' magazine, the Guernsey papers and Sark's Visitors' guide and several other magazines Ken knew. He then wrote a small brochure, and we decided what to charge and how many guests we could accommodate.

'I think only maximum of eight to start,' I insisted, although we had discussed turning three of the larger rooms into family rooms. They could easily take a set of bunk beds and a double. We calculated it would be possible to take twelve or thirteen people, but I was not ready even to think about that in our first year. Our plan was to encourage families and we had bought a small table tennis set and several games with the thought of rainy days and children needing entertainment. We even bought a colour television for guests' use in the lounge.

As the days stretched into weeks, I began to be a little nervous. We had only seen the place briefly on two occasions; I could not remember the colour scheme but had a suspicion it was mostly cream and green, too reminiscent of my hospital days. What cooking facilities were there? I had seen the old solid fuel Rayburn, but surely there had been a gas cooker too? How would we cope with a water supply dependant on a bore hole and rainwater? There was so much we did not know, and I was beginning to agree with friends we had lost our reason.

On top of this I was supposed to cook for guests who were expecting, according to Ken's brochure, 'good home cooked meals.' I had always loved cooking, being an 'intuitive' rather than 'stick to the recipe' type so hoped that would be acceptable. To settle my nerves, I started to plan a few menus, delving into several 'Good

Housekeeping' leaflets, eventually devising fourteen different ones, and experimented on Ken mostly to his delight.

Mr and Mrs Morris were a great help and sent a few instructions about our arrival, which we had planned for that February, 1966.

'Make sure you pack everything in the smaller British Rail 'A' containers, which can be shipped straight to Sark and they are small enough to get under the arch at the Maseline Harbour.' We knew they were talking about the more recent deep-water harbour built facing the North East, as opposed to the older 'Creux Harbour' which dried out in low tide and faced the other way and had been the access for centuries. 'If you have the bigger containers the carter will have to unpack everything at the harbour and carry it up bit by bit. I would also suggest you have a set each of cutlery, plates, and cup with you in your luggage. At that time of year the winds get up and sometimes boats are delayed. It could be a while before everything arrives.'

We were to bless that small piece of advice.

3/3

The day arrived to leave London and catch the train to Weymouth where we would board the overnight ferry to Guernsey. All our worldly goods, except two large suitcases and hand luggage had been packed in three British Rail containers and shipped to a warehouse in Southampton, where they would remain to be conveyed to Sark, via Guernsey.

I looked back at my first home as a married woman, from the taxi we had agreed as a necessary luxury, and I felt a little sad. We had some good times there; inviting the youth club members for impromptu parties and redecorating most of the rooms. Now we were off to a whole new experience and at a time when the weather was at its most unpleasant. Flurries of sleet greeted us as we arrived at the docks, and I looked with foreboding at the white capped waves. We had to move at that time of year to be organised in time for our first guests at Easter at the beginning of April.

'Ken, maybe we should have booked a sleeping cabin?'

'It is so much more expensive, and the seating is comfortable, Chris. You'll be alright.'

'It's OK for you. You could sleep anywhere.'

As soon as we hit the rough seas of the English Channel, I curled up in my chair and tried not to think how mad I was to be moving to an island where the only means of departure was by sea; I was a poor sailor at the best of times, but it was too late to worry about that now.

I must have dozed a little, but the night seemed endless, and my optimism reached the bottom rung. By the time we arrived in St Peter Port in Guernsey, I was thoroughly depressed as we disembarked onto the quay into the light of a new day. Everything was grey and waterlogged as we stood with our cases. Other passengers had been met or dispersed and we knew we had a couple of hours before the Sark boat was due to leave. As we stowed our cases in the left luggage shed, I grabbed my husband's arm.

'Oh, Ken I hope we are not making a big mistake.' I was near to tears with the lack of sleep.

'Come on, look there's a cafe sign just down there. What you need is a hot cup of tea and a good breakfast; you'll be alright.'

At the thought of fried food I felt sick again, but followed Ken into the warm welcoming cafe a little further down the quay. It was full of workmen and hummed with the Island patois which sounded like French but which I could not understand, though my French was quite good. With the warmth, a strong cup of tea and a plate of toast I was feeling a little better and my optimism returned a little. As there was still an hour to wait before the Sark boat departed, Ken and I decided to explore the nearer area of St Peter Port, the main town in Guernsey, and were lucky to find a small general store open, so I suggested we buy a few items. 'We'd better get some basic food for the next day or so; I don't know what we can get in Sark.' Loaded with a shopping bag each we set off towards the Sark departure quay which was right at the far end of the pier, of course. The wind blew straight into our faces as we battled to the steps which we would have to descend to step onto the deck. Our cases had been passed down by a crew member, and I was grateful for the strong grip of his calloused hand to guide me, as there was no handrail.

'Morning, Miss. Bit choppy today. You going down t'the cabin. eh?'

'Thanks for your help, but no thanks; I heard it called 'the Coffin.'

He laughed, 'Well y'do need t'have a strong stomach, *tu sais.*'

The boat we were travelling on was normally used for cargo and the small passenger cabin with no windows, was down a runged ladder. It did have a small bar so passengers could smoke and drink themselves to oblivion, but I had no intention of going down. There were a couple of benches up on the top deck, and that was where I told Ken I was going to stay.

'You'll get soaked. Well, I'm going down, anyway.'

'What about your asthma?'

'I'll be OK I have my puffer if I need it. Hang on tight up there, you don't want to be washed overboard!'

I climbed up the couple of steps to the small upper deck and settled down behind a box which I think held life jackets. I was glad I had put on my raincoat for as we sailed out of the harbour, spray found its way to my hiding place and my ponytail was soon soaked and my spectacles misted. I did not care, as my spirits rose while a shaft of weak sunlight lit up the pretty harbour and houses of St Peter Port. Peeping round my protection, I could see the islands of Herm and Jethou to the left, and way on the horizon the hump of Sark, looking like a basking whale. If I had fresh air, and there was plenty of that, I knew I would not feel sick, so settled to enjoy the rise and fall over the green churning seas.

Gradually Sark grew nearer, and we were soon passing the small white lighthouse at the end of the headland called *L'Epequerie,* and heading for Le Maseline harbour. The waters were a little calmer here as the inlet was sheltered, but the boat was still bumping up and down and it was impossible to put out the gangplank.

'You'll have t'jump miss. I'll tell y'when.' The crew member who had helped me in Guernsey, now held my elbow as I felt the deck heave up and down. As it lined up with the solid stone small quay, he said; 'Now, Miss' and propelled me into the arms of a young man standing waiting to help. As I untangled myself, and thanked him, I saw Ken waiting to take a leap and started up the granite steps to the upper quay. I knew there was a huge tidal variant...something like twenty-five feet...so sometimes the boat would line up with the steps and sometimes with the top quay. We were at the bottom of the steps so I was glad our suitcases, shopping and bags were handed up for us and we did not have to carry them ourselves.

As I reached the top, I looked around at the towering cliffs and grey landscape and my heart sank again.

Our visits had all been in May, when the wildflowers covered the cliffs, and the sea was calm and the sky blue. Now clouds threatened rain again and the rough cliffs were forbidding, and I realised this Island was so different from the Arcadian dream we had held. I waited as Ken arrived up the steps, wheezing a little from the effort.

'Oh, Ken! What have we done? How are we going to survive this? And more importantly, how do we get to 'Le Clos des Camps' with our luggage. That harbour hill is so steep.'

'There is the carter Jim, over there, we used when we were on holiday. He'll take the cases in his tractor trailer, I'm sure.'

'I don't think I could walk up the hill in this.' It had started to rain again.

Ken walked over to the red bearded Sarkee we had met before, and chatted for a moment, then beckoned to me.'

'Jim will take us to the top of the hill and deliver our cases. He can't take us any further than the Bel Air, though as it is against the law to carry passengers on the roads.'

Gratefully I clambered over the side of the tractor trailer, glad I had worn trousers, and sat on my suitcase just in time as Jim set off at full throttle, which he maintained all the way up the steep hill to the Pub at the top.

'Her y'are. Can't go no further. Bring the cases later.'

We thanked him and picked up our shopping and hand baggage as he disappeared into the bar and we turned to face the rain and started to tramp through the muddy roads to our new home.

3/4

Sark as a car-free Island was a welcome novelty when we were on holiday; faced with a mile long walk in drizzling rain in clothing not really suited to the conditions, was a different story.

We arrived at Clos des Camps dejected and cold, and I realised we had no key to let us in. We need not have worried, as the front door was not locked, and we were able to walk straight into a wonderfully warm house.

The Morris's had been in before us and lit the Rayburn.

I was almost in tears again at their kindness, and then noticed a covered tray on the kitchen table we had bought from the Morris' along with a couple of kitchen chairs and some other furniture.

'Oh, look Ken, they've left some scones, tea and a little milk. Aren't people kind.'

We sat in the warm kitchen, munching scones and enjoying the first cup of tea in our new home as I looked round the kitchen. My heart sank a little as my memory had been correct; green and cream paintwork and green and cream lino tiles. I also noticed the only other cooking facility, besides the Rayburn, were two gas rings. How on earth was I going to give 'good home cooking?'

Well, I had a few weeks to sort that before the first guests arrived at Easter.

I took the cups to wash over to the solid stone Butler sink with its wooden draining board, which I had not noticed when we bought the place and was grateful at least we had hot water from the Rayburn. It was a pity the sink was facing one of the walls and gave no view at all, but I supposed I would not have much time to gaze at anything anyway while I was washing guest's crockery.

Just as I had fished there was a sudden shrieking whistle from the front of the house.

'What on earth was that?' Ken walked quickly towards the noise, with me following close behind.

'Look, the wind is coming through the keyhole and making that noise. We'll have to put something over it; even if we don't have a key.' He stood in the entrance porch while I stayed in the hallway, which saved me from another soaking. The rain had set in again, and as Ken turned to join me a small stream of water seeped through the porch ceiling and dripped onto his head.

I should not have laughed but could not resist it at the sight of his expression and water dripping off his beard, though I admit it had a slightly hysterical note.

We had bought some towels and linen also from the Morris', so Ken dried quickly. We discovered later, when the porch had been added the gutter from the roof had just been left as it was, so flowed through the ceiling, spilling over when overloaded. When we rebuilt the porch much later, that and the whistling keyhole were put right.

For a while I wandered around the various rooms, becoming more and more despondent as there was little character to them. As the building was prefabricated, the walls were constructed in panels of particle board, like thick cardboard joined by strips of wood. This gave almost a temporary feeling to the rooms, and I wondered how we could make them more attractive. It was all so different from our high-ceilinged London flat with solid plastered walls.

As I looked in the lounge, I realised our lovely grey brocade curtains would clash with the existing decor, but I was pleased to see an attractive open fireplace. It was a pleasant room for all that, with a glass panelled door leading into the sunroom. I stepped down into this area we had decided to use as the dining room, and I could see its potential. A low wall reached to about waist height, with a shallow shelf all around. Above that was all glass, consisting of many small windows...I counted about fifty...and above that a sloping roof. There was another half glass door at the far end which led outside by the back door and a rough lawn. It had obviously been added to the original house, as the two large casement windows in the kitchen opened into the sunroom. I tapped on one to attract Ken's attention as he was busy unpacking the shopping bags, and he opened it.

'Hello. Are you having fun, exploring?'

I grimaced a little. 'Lot of repainting needed, but I think it will be convenient to be able to hand things through the window to serve the tables, don't you agree?'

Apart from the paintwork, which would be possible to change, the overall feeling of the place was beginning to grow on me. I had to admit the pelting rain and grey clouds would have depressed anyone, and my usual optimism began to return as we sat in the kitchen eating chunks of bread and cheese from out Guernsey shopping.

'You know, Ken, I am sure there will be the possibility to look after a patient here in the winter. Mrs Morris said people had to be sent to Guernsey if they were taken ill. You know, a stroke or something?'

'Well, I'm not sure. Guests come first.'

'No-one will come in winter.'

'You never know: workmen and such.'

'I don't think I want workmen with muddy boots and clothes...'

'We'll see...'

Although all our energies had been put into getting the guest house business going, I was still determined to nurse on Sark. I had not trained all that time to abandon my chosen profession.

As the afternoon wore on, there was still no sign of our luggage, and we were becoming a little anxious.

'I wonder if we can ring someone. Maybe he's taken it to the wrong place?'

We both looked at the antiquated telephone receiver on the wall. It was a long brown wooden box with a handle at one side and a Bakelite receiver resting on a hook at the other side. While staying on holiday we had used a similar one, but we had been supervised and I for one could not remember exactly what to do.

'I think you just wind that handle and lift the receiver: I remember we were told the telephonist answers and knows all that is going on ...'

'You can't just ask her where our cases are!'

'It's worth a try.' I wound the handle and quickly snatched the Bakelite receiver from its hook. For a moment there was a crackle and then a loud voice nearly made me drop it.

'Good afternoon, Mrs Davies; welcome to Sark. Mrs West here, and what can I do for you?'

'Er, Um; thank you. We were wondering if it was possible to trace our luggage...'

'I think your carter will be Jim Le Feuvre...I expect he is still in the Bel Air...leave it with me.'

Within a half hour we heard the roar of a tractor in the road outside, and saw our carter unload our cases by the gate, and off he went up the road.

'Good job the rain's stopped,' muttered Ken as he put on his waterproof and went to collect them.

I was very impressed with out telephone service and realised life on Sark was going to be full of new and unexpected experiences as I went to help Ken with the cases. The telephone exchange was a hub of information, and I was to learn it was seldom necessary to know anyone's phone number, as we would be put in touch with whoever we were trying to contact.

The cases were a little damp on the outside, and I was glad we had lined them inside with plastic, so the contents were still dry as we unpacked in one of the bedrooms at the front. The wardrobes were all built in, and as we had bought a double bed from the Morris' it seemed the best place to spend our first night.

'It's a bit cold in here.' Ken was wheezing a little with the damp air, 'we must remember to leave the kitchen and bedroom doors open...it will be a bit like central heating. Why don't we drag the mattress into the kitchen for tonight?'

It was quite easy to do that, and we set it before the warm Rayburn, and so that was how we spent our first cosy night in our new home.

3/5

The sun streaming through the windows from the conservatory woke me and I sat up for a moment wondering where I was. Ken was still sound asleep by my side, so I rolled off the mattress and pulled myself up by the rail on the Rayburn, enjoying the warmth still glowing from it. My first reaction to the solid cooker had been 'the sooner that goes the better,' and I had dubbed it 'the Monstrosity' thinking of trying to cook on it and the bother of having to stoke it all the time with messy coal. I was now beginning to give it a second chance: it was so comforting to have constant warmth. In London we had a series of electric heaters, and had packed some to join us in Sark, but here had always been the delay until they warmed up a room. I also discovered later that as the electricity was mostly generated on the island and dependant on expensively imported oil, the cost was about eight times as much as we had paid in London, so use of electrical goods was strictly limited.

I patted the rail; 'Well, we'll see what you cook like...'

Ken opened his eyes and peered over the top of the bedclothes. 'Who are you talking to, Chris?'

'Er; just myself. Would you like a cuppa? The kettle is warm and won't take a moment.' That was another good thing; the big solid kettles constantly on the cooker top always seemed near to boiling so it only took a minute to finish them on the gas ring. Dressing quickly, we had our breakfast...Ken had of course bought some *'All bran'* in Guernsey...and I could not wait to go outside to see our home properly.

'I'd better stoke up the fire first.' Ken had been shown by Mr Morris the ritual of filling the coal shuttle from the bunker outside the night before, so it would be ready in the morning to keep the fire going. The Morris' had done this for us, as we had not given it a thought. Gingerly Ken opened the fire door, to be met with a blast of hot air and a few sparks flying onto the floor tiles, which he quickly stamped out. He slammed the door and then remembered he had to open the damper fully at the base of the chimney, first. The second try was more successful, though his aim in swinging the long shuttle to throw the coal into the firebox took many tries over the next few weeks to be perfected, without a fair mount ending on the kitchen floor.

At last we were ready to explore.

'I think I'll just wander round the boundaries and look at the state of the fields.'

'The fields;' I could hardly believe all this lovely rich green land surrounding us was ours. So much time and energy had been taken with planning the guest house, I had not given much thought to the land.

The sky was a pale blue with scarcely a cloud in sight, and I was to learn this was a peculiarity of these islands surrounded by sea. Conditions changed overnight, from wind and rain to a wonderful clear skies and sunshine...and the reverse.

For a while I explored the large front garden, if you could call the few lupine trees and hydrangeas bordered by a high privet hedge a garden. The grass was quite long, and I remembered we had been told there was an old mower in the corrugated iron shed in the far corner of our field next to the bungalow. As soon as it was dry the lawn would need to be cut.

I wandered round to the back and delighted in the open vista and sight of the two fields which we owned. They looked to be good grass, bordered on the boundaries by waist high banks, much as I had seen in Cornwall on a holiday. I later learned this protection from salty winds was vital. Anything which was exposed to the burning blasts soon withered and died.

Overcome by delight at having our very own bit of Sark, my heart lifted with pure joy and I could not stop myself flinging full length on the ground tearing up a couple of tufts of grass and throwing them in the air, shouting; 'It's ours! It's all ours!'

A fruity chuckle behind me made me scramble up and turn to see the weather-beaten face of Hap, a Sarkee we had met on holiday at the old farmhouse, peering over the bank.

'Buggre; you ploughing by hand then, eh?'

I laughed and tried to hide my blush. I had taken an instant liking to this middle-aged farmer and we had developed a rapport when we had met before: something which I was later to discover was unusual between the indigenous Sarkese of Norman French extraction, and the English residents. Hap was the quintessential farmer with his cap set at a slight angle, face burned ruddy by working in all weathers, and a twinkle in his blue eyes.

'Welcome then Mrs Chris. Any chance of a 'wet', eh?'

I knew what he meant and invited our first guest into the kitchen for a cup of tea, quickly washing up the only beakers we had. I wondered how long it would be before all our other belongings arrived as all we had were the two cups lent us and two sets we had packed in our suitcases.

I remembered Hap had a sweet tooth and was glad we had bought a sticky treacle cake and offered him a slice.

I gestured to the Rayburn; 'Hope I can manage that thing to cook you a proper cake one day.'

'Good thing those; we got one. Got to watch the wind though. Blows one way and it burns, and the other no heat at all, eh? You settling alright then?'

'We've only been in one night.'

'Cosy though, eh?' He glanced at the mattress, and I blushed again.

'It was so cold and wet last night.'

'Where's your man, then?' He seldom called Ken by name, and there was always more of a reserve with him. Before I answered, he continued. 'You planning to grow potatoes? Cos if y'are ye need to get em in soon, eh?'

I smiled to myself and remembered how I had been intrigued when I had first heard the Islanders' way of speaking, with a Gaelic twang and ending most sentences almost as a question.

'I don't know. You'll need to talk to Ken.'

'What about the nursing, then? You still planning?'

'I hope so. Hap we've only just arrived as I said!'

'We need a nurse. Well I'll leave y'to it. I look forward to those cakes, eh?' With that he clapped his cap back on covering the two-tone line on his brow, baby white where it had been covered and dark brown from many summer suns.

I watched as he climbed the bank, not realising my life would be bound up with this man and his family for many years to come, and that they would become my 'Sark Family.'

When Ken returned later he was delighted with his exploration. 'It looks good fertile land, Chris. We can grow vegetables I am sure, maybe a few potatoes and so on.'

'That reminds me, Hap called in and asked if we were going to grow potatoes...'

'What was he doing here?'

'I just said; he was sort of passing and called to welcome us and asked if we were going to grow potatoes.'

'Why would he ask that?'

'Maybe he is offering help? I seem to remember his family have a shop in the village and he runs a farm, doesn't he? You could call in maybe and ask?'

Ken said nothing and I realised it would have to be me, doing the asking. Ken was not one to push himself forward. I had met May, Hap's wife, and his daughter Annie when I had occasionally visited their general grocery shop while on holiday. They had treated me with the quiet reserve meted out to English residents. His son in law, Sam, I had also met as I collected milk for Mr and Mrs French from the farm they worked, and he had been a little more friendly, being a Guernsey man and more used to 'Foreigners.'

Hap and Sam rented the farm belonging to the Seigneurie, the home of the Dame and current ruler of the Island and it was just across the road from our new home. I was not sure if I should go over and look for Hap there or go to the store in the village but decided to postpone that for a few days. We had more important things to do.

3/6

The weather stayed fine for a while, with just the strong wind to contend with. This meant the cargo boat could not bring our railway containers from Guernsey as the rough seas in the Maseline harbour made it impossible for the boat to tie up. Smaller items were manhandled ashore, but we just had to wait. We had been told one of the containers was still in Southampton in any case.

'I do hope they come before you go back to London, Ken.' Time was running out and Ken would soon be returning to London for a few weeks, leaving me on my own.

A few days after my conversation with Hap, I walked to the village and called in at his family store. Annie, his daughter was behind the counter, and I could see she was pregnant. I knew she had two young children already and wondered how women managed on this little Island with only one doctor and no midwife: I assumed Annie would have to go to Guernsey.

I was to discover differently.

As expected, Hap was at the farm, but I chatted a little with Annie and bought a few items and asked where we could buy milk.

'Oh, I'll get my husband Sam to deliver if you like. Do you have a can or covered jug? We don't have bottles here, eh.!'

When I said we didn't have anything like that, she said to wait a moment, and returned with a couple of two-pint metal cans with handles and lids.

'You can have these if you like; be sure to scald them out with boiling water.'

I knew the milk on the Island was not pasteurised although TT tested. It was from the Guernsey cattle which gave rich creamy milk fresh from the cows, each morning. The farmers were only allowed to have this particular breed, so all the milk would be unadulterated by less rich milk.

Annie was a typical reserved Sark woman, but as she was about my age she was more relaxed with the English residents than the older generation were. She came from one of the older families who had been the first settlers four hundred years ago, as of course was her father, Hap.

After we chatted for a while, I asked her when her baby was due.

'In May: but I tell you one thing, eh. I'm not going to Guernsey to have it, for sure.'

'Is that what women usually do?'

'Sometimes: but I told that new Doctor King. I'm not going, so there.' She thought for a moment then said; 'You're a nurse aren't you? You can help him, eh?'

I did not want to get involved with that discussion so picked up the cans and my purchases and said goodbye quickly as someone else had come into the shop and Annie turned to serve them. I was not a midwife and in fact had never seen a baby born, although as a district nurse I had been shown emergency delivery films.

After walking home and leaving my purchases at Le Clos des Camps and wishing the container with our bikes would arrive soon, I wandered across the road to the Seigneurie farm. There was a wooded valley leading down to a stony beach called Port du Moulin just a little way along, and access to the farm was through a grove of oak trees to the left of the path. I had been surprised when first visiting this wind-battered Island to discover there were several sheltered valleys, lushly wooded and carpeted with wildflowers in summer. Now of course the trees were bare, but I was delighted to see a few primroses already peeping through the thick grass as I followed the path to the farm buildings.

I could hear voices in a barn, one unmistakably Hap's so headed in that direction. Just as I arrived the man himself appeared and gave me a big grin.

'Morning Mrs Chris. You bringing me a slice of your cake, eh?'

The young man who followed I recognised as Annie's husband Sam, and he nodded to me while raising an eyebrow at his father-in-law. I expect he was not used to the way Hap spoke to me, but I just laughed. 'Not mastered the Monstrosity yet, but can I talk to you about potatoes?'

'You want us to plant eh? We do it by machine. I'll show ye.' He took me into one of the barns and he pointed to a hopper type of trailer with a couple of seats placed either side, and a couple of plough tines below.

'You put the seed potatoes in the hopper and you and your man sit there and drop them down the chute. I'll be towing it in the tractor and they'll be ploughed in. Mind, you must make sure potatoes are the right way up, eh?'

I started to say, 'How do you know...' than caught he twinkle in Hap's eye and saw Sam was trying not to grin. I shook my head and had to admit I had walked into that one.

We made a time for the planting, and Hap said he would supply the potatoes.

'Usually Aron Pilot for earlies and you'll need some later ones. Leave it t'me. I'll come and plough the day before, eh?'

I hurried back to find Ken who was in the green shed at the far corner of our big field next to the bungalow. He was looking at the old petrol motor mower we had bought with the property.

'Not sure how good this will be. Maybe you could have a go while I'm away? It's a pity I will be leaving soon, but you'll be alright, won't you?'

It was the first time he had said anything about his departure since we had arrived, and I was touched Ken had obviously been a little concerned. He was not a demonstrative man, and I knew his strict Methodist upbringing had squashed any spontaneity he might have had. It was this which had contributed to a near breakdown when he was in his early twenties. He had told me the combination of studying for exams, his journalistic responsibilities for a local paper and a disastrous love affair had had a heavy toll and he just collapsed at work one day. He also said he had a twin who had died at birth, and for a while as a child he had thought his parents were not his. For about eighteen months he had attended a psychiatrist for consultations, and this had restored his equilibrium, but had not added to his slight feeling of inferiority.

On the appointed day Hap rolled up with his tractor after softening the ground the day before with a deep ploughing. The weather had turned cold and windy again, and having been warned by Hap we were muffled up in warm clothing. Even so it was a freezing job as we sat balanced on the two flat backless seats by the hoppers pushing small seed potatoes down the chutes. After the first row, Hap stopped and brought us a couple of old sacs.

'Here, sit on these. You don't want piles, eh?' That did help a little as the wind had been whistling through the holes in the bottom of the seats adding to our discomfort.

At last the potatoes were planted and we staggered to our warm kitchen inviting Hap to join us for a 'wet.' I was beginning to appreciate the comfort of the old 'Monstrosity,' Rayburn.

Within a couple of days the wind had dropped again and we were pleased as we had decided to go over to Guernsey on the 'Wednesday Shopping Trip.' This weekly boat left its berth in St Peter Port harbour in Guernsey at eight in the morning and returned at nine from Sark to Guernsey. It was the one day of the week (except for once a month on a Saturday, weather permitting) when Sark residents could go to Guernsey and return on the same day. The return from Guernsey to Sark set off at three fifteen.

I needed to have a good look at the main store, Creasey's, in St Peter Port while Ken wanted to visit and sign up with a warehouse which supplied wholesale goods to guest houses and hotels. First most of the residents who had braved the trip made a bee-line for a favourite cafe, Maison Carre in St Peter Port's main shopping street, Le Pollet. As we trooped in the waitresses smiled, regarding our windswept hair, serviceable laced shoes and all-weather gear and remarked; 'I see the Sark boat's in.'

Fortified by a strong cup of coffee and a toasted teacake Ken and I parted our ways, agreeing to meet up for lunch at the same cafe at one o'clock. I spent a happy couple of hours browsing through the departments of Creasey's and then going to the wonderful covered market where fruit, vegetables, meat, and bread stalls offered their wares. There was such a milling of people and hustle and bustle I felt like a country bumpkin after only a few weeks on Sark. I wondered how I had ever survived in London.

After a lunch together, Ken said he had something else to do and we agreed to meet up at the quay at three. I was quite happy to return to Creasey's, where I had seen some pretty bedspreads which I thought would brighten up the bedrooms.

I arrived at the quay in good time but there was no sign of my usually punctual husband. Just as I was starting to worry, he arrived a little breathless to help me load the shopping onto the ferry, and I noticed a large bulge in the pocket of his 'Army surplus' duffle coat.

As he sat heavily next to me, a small black nose followed by a silvery head peeped out of his pocket.

'Ken, what on earth...?'

'Well, I thought you might be lonely with me gone.'

'Oh, he's a darling. What shall we call him?' I asked as I cuddled the tiny Labrador puppy.

That was how 'Hugo' came into our lives.

3/7

The fine weather held and at last two of our containers arrived in time for Ken to help unpack, but the one stuck in Southampton had carpets and most of the crockery and cutlery in it. We had decided to bring our lovely grey carpet from London and replace the rather lively patterned one in the lounge, as it would match our Italian brocade curtains but of course we had a problem there as I complained to Ken.

'We will just have to leave the furniture piled in the lounge until the container arrives. I sure Sam will help me.' I just hoped all would be sorted before our first guests arrived.

I was sad to see Ken go but not as bereft as I feel I should have been to see my husband depart after only a few years of marriage. I was also a little incensed he was happy to do this but reminded myself we needed all the money we could scrape together, and a tax refund would be most welcome.

I had to admit to a slight feeling also of relief not to be sharing my bed for a few weeks. I had not become used to this, even after five years, and what I had expected to be an exciting sexual experience, had mostly left me frustrated. While I was still a virgin when I married, I had indulged in what was then called 'heavy petting' with one or two boyfriends before I was married and had expected this sort of thing as foreplay with Ken. It was not so; even his kissing was a closed lip peck. When I had once tried French kissing, which I had been excited to learn, he pulled back with surprise and dislike. I had discovered I enjoyed sex and had been looking forward to married life where the restrictions would be removed. I had now learned not every relationship promised fulfilment in that respect, so my energies began to be channelled elsewhere.

I had a great deal to do before our first guests arrived at Easter just five weeks away. Bookings had been quite good; mainly thanks to Ken's attractive wording on our advertisements and brochure. The first guests to arrive would be a family of three from Holland, and they were staying for a full two weeks. I only hoped my cooking would be good enough. The Monstrosity and I had come to an understanding and most of the time it behaved itself, but it did depend which direction the wind blew, as Hap had warned us. A stiff North Easter fanned the fire into a raging inferno if not damped down, and a gentle wet South Wester needed chiding and cajoling to boil even a kettle.

I had a list of jobs to do but still in the back of my mind was a plan to nurse on Sark. A new doctor had arrived not long before we did, and I thought it a good idea to strike while the iron was hot and introduce myself. First I thought I had better visit the retired nurse who had been working with the previous doctor.

I knew she had been married to one of the Sarkees, but had retired from the hospital in Guernsey after his death.

The cottage was a typical Island dwelling; made of granite and painted white. The roof would have been thatched years ago, but now had corrugated iron which I felt spoiled its picturesque appearance. For the rest, the roses round the door just showing the first green leaves, and a jumbled bed of wallflowers, primulas and violets by the solid wooden door made up for the unattractive roof.

The door was ajar and I knocked timidly. I had rung earlier asking if I might call, and the firm voice at the other end of the phone called to mind a few nursing sisters I had known. She was tall and thin, with her grey hair scraped into an old-fashioned bun at the nape of her neck, but the welcome was friendly enough. She offered me a cup of tea, which I accepted, then, as we sat in comfortable chintz covered armchairs she said

'I understand you want to nurse here, Mrs Davies?'

'Well, I would like to, but I was told you have been working with the previous doctor...?'

She waved her hand dismissively; 'You are welcome if the Dame agrees.' At my raised eyebrows she continued,

'You have been to see Dame Sybil Hathaway?'

'Er, well no.'

'There's not much goes on here that she is not involved in. I would suggest you make an appointment as soon as you can. She usually vets most new residents anyway.'

As I made my departure, I was a little bemused. I knew the 'ruler' of Sark was an elderly woman who had inherited the title from her father, there not being a male heir. She was well known as a strong-willed woman in her late seventies and had saved the Island from total devastation by the German occupying forces during the Second World War. That I should need to see her had not occurred to me, and the thought made me a little nervous. I supposed she was regarded as 'Royalty' on the Island and I was not comfortable with how I should behave.

On return home I felt there was no time like the present and asked the telephone exchange to connect me to the Seigneurie, the home of Dame Hathaway. Expecting a housekeeper to answer, I was taken aback when a strong very well-spoken voice answered my call, and I realised it was the Dame herself.

'Ah yes,' was her reply after I had introduced myself, 'you are the new people at Le Clos des Camps, aren't you? Come to afternoon tea tomorrow; say three fifteen.'

There was an assumption I would be free which irritated me a little, but then I guessed Dame Sybil was used to being obeyed. In any case it was a necessary step if I wanted to follow my dream of nursing on Sark.

To say I was not nervous on walking through the wrought iron gates and down the gravel drive towards the beautifully proportioned Seigneurie house, would not have been accurate, but I was determined not to be cowed. As I pulled the ornate handle for the bell, I quickly straightened my jacket and took a deep breath. After all I had faced austere Matrons in my time, not to mention a few of the wealthy dental customers in London.

The door was opened by a middle-aged woman who I rightly guessed was the housekeeper. She nodded to me as I said my name and ushered me through a door to the right of the main entrance. As I followed her, I had a glimpse of a long, polished table to my left in what appeared to be a dining room, and wide stairs leading up the side of the large room.

'Would you wait in here please, Mrs Davies.'

It was cosy, with a fire blazing in the hearth and comfortable chairs with a small wooden coffee table in front. A rich rug: I supposed Persian, added luxury as did the pictures of horses and dogs on the walls and china ornaments on the mantle. While I was wondering if I should sit down or stay standing, the door opened again and the regal figure of Dame Sybil Hathaway entered, leaning lightly on her walking stick.

'Good afternoon Mrs Davies; do sit down.' She was all I had expected of this legendary lady. I had heard stories of how she had faced the German officers during the occupation with her ability to speak fluently in German. She had spent some time in that country before the war, and because of that, had managed to make life bearable for the residents. I could see the firmness of jaw and bright intelligent eyes behind her spectacles and knew La Dame was still in total command.

The door opened again and the housekeeper entered, setting a loaded tea tray onto the coffee table, and left.

'Perhaps you would pour, Mrs Davies. Just a little milk and no sugar, please.'

I was glad of something to do, and managed without spilling anything, and handed the fragile bone china cup and saucer to Dame Sybil. I served myself and tackled a sandwich, hoping I would not drop crumbs on the Persian rug.

'And how are you settling in, Mrs Davies?'

I mumbled a reply, trying not to speak with my mouth full, and we conversed with trivialities until we had both finished.

'Now, I understand you want to act as a district nurse here?' She picked up a letter which had been lying on a small table by her side. 'I have had this letter from the Queen's Institute of District Nurses in London, where I believe you were last practicing?' She looked over her spectacles at me, 'they said they were delighted I would be having a district nurse here at last, but I knew nothing of it of course, as you had not informed me of your intent...until now.'

With face flushing, I felt like a first-year nurse in front of the matron for a misdemeanour but kept my cool. I did not want to cross this formidable person, but I was not going to apologise either.

Dame Sybil stood up, 'Well I am sure the English residents will be glad of your help, but I doubt if you will have any Sarkese patients, Mrs Davies.'

I was dismissed.

But Dame Sybil was to be proved very wrong.

3/8

After my visit to La Dame, I decided my next step was to see the doctor and rang to make an appointment to have a chat. I discovered his home and surgery were both in a large house near an old windmill at the highest point in the Island. Having been united at last with my trusty 'Moulton' bike which had arrived in one of the containers, I was able to cycle to the doctor's house.

I puffed my way up the steep hill and stopped to get my breath back at the top, and had a proper look at the Mill. It belonged to the Island ruler and in years gone by people could have their grain milled, but a small tithe was charged. I had been told the blades were removed years ago, and I saw the mechanism was still visible on the grass by its side. I thought it a pity it was not still whole, like the ones I had seen in visits to my brother in Holland. I then discovered a small cottage had been built attached to one rounded wall, so the blades would not have been able to turn in any case.

I propped my bike against the wall by the doctor's house, wondering if I needed to lock it, but decided not to: after all most people on Sark did not even lock their houses. The surgery was housed in a small extension at one side of the charming two-story building, and I debated with myself whether I should go to the front door or not, but the decision was made for me by a cheery call from a man working in a flowerbed to one side.

'Hello, there. You must be Mrs Davies? You've arrived in the nick of time.'

He was a man of about fifty, with a red face and a fringe of hair round a balding head. He made me think of a monk of old, with his twinkling eyes and jolly smile, and I thought: 'I shall enjoy working with you.'

Dr King wiped his hands on a handkerchief from his pocket and offered his hand for me to shake, which I did. 'I'm sure it is time for elevenses. Come and meet the little woman.' I smiled to myself at the use of a name for the morning tea, which was a favourite of my dear father. It brought a small lump to my throat when I thought of all the times we had enjoyed a cup of coffee and his favourite 'club' chocolate biscuits at 'elevenses time'.

Mrs King was indeed little, and I smiled at her as she ushered us into the sitting room at the front of the house. Everything about her was small and neat, from a perfectly curled hairstyle to her small feet encased in pretty leather shoes.

'Come in, my dears, I will bring in the coffee...'

Dr King surprised me by telling his wife to sit, and he would get the coffee. 'I need to wash my hands anyway.'

Mrs King... 'Call me Dulce,'...sat as she was told but shook her head. 'My dear Robert fusses so. I had malaria in Jamaica where we lived for many years...he was a doctor there, you know. But I am quite better now.' She stifled a cough, and I was concerned at the slight wheeze afterwards but said nothing.

The coffee and biscuits arrived, and as Dr King handed me a beaker, asked what I wanted to discuss with him.

'Well, I am a qualified district nurse, and I was wondering if it would be all right for me to practice here?'

'Most certainly, young woman: I would be delighted. Er, you have been to see Dame Sybil I assume?'

I looked at the doctor and raised my eyebrows and nodded. 'Yes, indeed I have.'

'Did you have the third degree, then?' Dulce asked, with a smile.

'Not exactly,' and I told them what had happened. 'I'm afraid I got off on the wrong foot. I had no idea the QIDN would write to her like that.'

Dulce patted my knee. 'Don't worry dear. She only wants what is best for the Island, and I am sure Robert will be glad of your help, won't you dear?'

'I certainly will. It's strange not to have other doctors to discuss patients with. I have always been with a clinic group before, and of course here I must supply the medications as well as prescribe them.' He went on to explain his full responsibilities.

I began to feel a little sorry for anyone who took on this post. Besides being the sole medical practitioner, I understood he would be the Medical Officer of Health, and as there was not a vet on the Island either, some animal husbandry as well.

'It is not at all what I am used to, but we'll see, we'll see.'

Within a year Dulce and Robert King left Sark for a busier practice in England, partly because of Dulce's failing health, but also, I suspected the professional isolation was too daunting.

Back home, I busied myself decorating the lounge in a silver-grey paint, which I thought would match the curtains. With a large round 'sunburst' rug in the middle of the room and some bright pictures, I was sure the room would be more attractive...just as soon as the final container arrived and I could get the two settees and armchairs in place.

I next tackled the kitchen, and although I could do nothing with the green and cream floor tiles, a bright white paint on the walls and ceiling, and buttercup yellow on the cupboard doors made everything much brighter. The bedrooms were all in a muted white, and as I had the bright bedcovers from Guernsey, I felt there was no need to do more there yet.

The early spring weather was warming the soil, and I just loved to be outside. Little puppy Hugo was great company: he was a mischievous scamp, but he was beginning to know his name and mostly came to my call...when he wanted to. I had him on a long piece of rope when I was working outside, after I had played 'throw' a while to tire him.

Having painted as much as I could inside, I next turned to the garden. While I knew Ken was planning to grow vegetables for the guests, I decided it would be a good idea to get a few sown as soon as possible, so I took another trip over to Guernsey to buy seeds. I was concerned to leave Hugo alone, but Sam took charge when he delivered the milk.

'I'll have him in the tractor cab with me Mrs Chris, if y'like. I've got the kids with me anyway.'

I was back by mid-afternoon, and I don't think Hugo had missed me at all, though I was happy to have my little companion back.

The next day, after chasing the puppy around to tire him and throwing a stick, I tied him up and set to planting carrots, leeks, beetroot and lettuce seeds, criss-crossing strands of string tied to marker stick to ward off birds and identify the rows of seeds.

A few days later I decided to try cutting the front lawn with the old petrol cylinder mower we had bought with the property. I knew a little about these machines as my father had one once, and I made sure it had oil and petrol in the right tanks. There was a lever at the side to engage and disengage the gear, and starting it was by pulling a chord on the engine. At about my fourth pull it spluttered into life much to my satisfaction. I had remembered to disengage the gear first.

All went well for a couple of rows, but I was having difficulty with the gear lever, as it was hard to pull. As I was trying the third trip down towards the flower bed near the road, the lever just jammed and the mower took off on its own, ploughing through the emerging daffodils and only stopping as it hit the bank and stalled. The jolt of the mower taking off threw me back onto my bottom and I sat there not sure whether to laugh or cry. As I was about to get up, I heard a small woof behind me and looked back to see Hugo. I had left him locked in the kitchen as I did not want to disturb him with the mower sounds. Somehow he had escaped, and looking at me with a wagging tail, he offered me a stake...attached to other stakes tied together with string.

My vegetable markers.

3/9

I had discovered the winter months on Sark brought few visitors and new residents were a source of general interest, especially in my case as my husband had gone off and left me to fend for myself.

I did not really have any near neighbours as we were surrounded by fields, but in such a small island no-one was very far away. I had also been visiting May and Annie's shop and the other larger store in the village, called 'The Bakery.' This store was a general hub for residents, as it not only sold the delicious home baked goods which gave its name, but also most groceries and a selection of vegetables. Here I had met and chatted to a few other women who lived on the Island.

One such was Sue de Carteret, the wife of the harbour master we had briefly met on our arrival. She was an interesting lady and spoke with a noticeable Canadian accent, which intrigued me, and she asked if she might call in some time. I was delighted of course, as being on my own with only Hugo to talk to had its limitations. I wanted to know more about my new home and hoped she would enlighten me.

Sue arrived with a gift of half a dozen eggs, and I invited her in and soon made a cup of coffee from the constantly simmering, solid bottomed kettle on the Rayburn hotplate.

I showed her into the lounge, where the furniture was scattered a little haphazardly, but at least it was warm as the fire was lit. The final container had arrived at last, and Sam and one of his farm workers had helped me unload, and he had promised to help sort the lounge, but I had to wait until he was free of farm duties to lay the carpet. Sue did not seem to mind, chatting in her attractive accent as she sipped her coffee and accepted my homemade rock cake.

'It's great to have fresh blood! A lot of the 'ex colonials'...we call the *"lower cocktail set"* ...go to the

Canary Islands or Spain for most of the winter.' She munched one of my cakes and I hoped it was not the texture suggestive of its name; I had not quite mastered cooking in the Monstrosity yet. She continued... 'we get bored with the same old faces.'

'What do you mean by *"lower cocktail set"*?'

She laughed: 'Well, there are really four social groups here. You can call them classes if you like,' she shrugged. 'There is the Dame and the very wealthy. They tend to socialise together; they are the *"upper cocktail set"*, then there are the *"lower cocktail set,"* who also have their own little group.' She drained her cup. 'Then there are the *"working English"*, like you and me...well I'm Canadian; and the *Sarkese*, who keep themselves to themselves.'

'Goodness, it sounds complicated. Do you mean they keep in their, er, groups?'

'Well, mostly. I am married to a *Sarkese*, so I run foul of both the *Sarkese* and the English.' She said it with a flippant tone, but I noted sadness in her tone, and was curious to discover more about this person who I hoped would become a friend. I learned she was a Canadian Professor of Anthropology who had travelled to Sark some years ago to study the local Sarkese; had fallen in love with one, and married him.

Through Sue I met several other women who ran guest houses or worked directly or indirectly in the tourist industry. Thinking it a good way of learning what made the Island tick, one day I invited a few ladies for afternoon tea. I had by then managed to produce passable scones and buns, and had the Rayburn stoked and the fire lit in the lounge. At last the carpet had been laid and the couch, bed settee and easy chairs put in place. I felt it all looked very cosy and hoped the others would be impressed and bear us in mind in the coming season as a referral if they were full. I had learned this was the standard practice among the guest houses and it was well worth making sure you were on the 'roster.'

All went well for a while until I went back into the kitchen to top up the teapot and refill the kettle: but there was no water in the tap. We had a borehole and an underground rainwater tank; I could not believe they were dry. Then I realised that the ancient pump which had been coughing and rattling away since we had moved in, had finally burned out, and the header tank in the loft was empty. With the Rayburn at full blast I had visions of the hot water tank exploding like a bomb. I realised the best thing I could do was damp down the fire, but that would be difficult. The alternative I realised was to transport the live coals to the fire in the lounge.

I popped my head round the lounge door. 'Excuse me ladies, I have a little problem; my blessed pump has packed up and I am worried about the Rayburn overheating the hot water cylinder, so I need volunteers to transfer the live coals to this fire.' I produced as many spades and shovels as I could find and amidst giggles and coughs, we transferred all the live coals. It was only as we finished, and there were just a few coals left in the Rayburn's fire box, Sue remarked, 'you know I am sure these stoves have a safety valve Chris, and can't empty if there is no water to feed in.' I looked blankly at her amid sighs and laughter among my departing guests. I realised this would probably do the rounds with some hilarity at my expense.

I knew the Island was a place for gossip and community stories, and I supposed it was a little like the children's "whispering game" where a whispered sentence was passes around the children at a party and in the end the first sentence bore no resemblance to the final one. This did not worry me as I had nothing to hide. I had once heard someone say 'well if they are talking about me, someone else is having a rest.' I was not sure how Ken would like this, as he was essentially a private person, but I did not expect he would socialise enough to be aware of any gossip.

Some of the stories made me realise how finely balanced the relationship between the 'incomers' and the Sarkese was. On one of his visits Hap related a story which emphasised this. He told me of a particular ex-colonial resident who stopped a local woman taking a short cut through his fields. She consequently missed the boat.

'What happened? Did the family complain?'

'Well no, not exactly,' he looked innocently at me.

'It was bad luck that the next day when they were unloading his laundry, it fell into the harbour, eh?'

I had several other visitors, some of whom were not as welcome. As in any community, there were one or two would be Casanovas who fancied their chances with anything in skirts. When it was known I was on my own, I received several phone calls and even visits from these gentlemen. I tactfully told them I was only awaiting my husband's return from settling our business, and no thanks I really did not want a lover. I suppose I was a little flattered, but not at all tempted. I mentioned this to Hap, one day, and his usual casual attitude changed.

'You leave it to me Mrs Chris. Can't have this: I'll have a word, eh?'

In some ways the grapevine proved advantageous, as the fact I was wanting to practice as a nurse in the community helped, and contrary to La Dame's prediction, my first patient was an old Sarkese lady.

The call came just as I was falling asleep after a tiring day sorting the contents of the third container of belongings.

'Is that the nurse? Doctor said to ring. Can you come and see to mother, please?' The voice was hesitant. 'The undertaker can't get over till tomorrow. I'll send a tractor for you: I have special permission from the Constable.' I could hardly say 'no' and was grateful I would not be trying to find the house in the dark on my bicycle. Normally no tractors were allowed out after ten at night without special permission.

Shivering, I changed back into thick trousers and sweater, boots and waterproof jacket. A draughty trip on the step of a tractor made me suitably subdued, but death had no worries for me. I gently washed the old Sark grandmother, dressing her in a special nightdress kept for the occasion. Popping in her false teeth and tucking a pillow under her jaw, to stop her mouth gaping, I straightening her arms. She looked so peaceful.

My first Sark patient.

3/10

Spring seemed just round the corner, with daffodils and primroses brightening every bank and the blackthorn looking like snow on the dark winter branches. The weather was milder but still strong winds sprang up from nowhere and I soon became used to it, but began to realise why people on the island always seemed to know what the weather forecast was. At first, I had been surprised, but when our cargo delivery, shopping trips and later our guests' arrival depended on the severity and direction of the wind, I became an expert also.

I knew if a strong northeast wind blew into the new 'Masiline' harbour, no boat could tie up there. The other, much older 'Creux' harbour, used for centuries by local fishermen and facing the opposite direction, was only usable during high tide, as it drained dry otherwise.

As Easter approached and my first guests were expected, I watched the forecast with anxiety, hoping my guests would not be stranded in Guernsey. Ken was not due back until the week afterwards, and so I had the anxiety of making sure everything was working and ready, on my own. The new pump had been installed soon after my disastrous afternoon tea and I was reasonably confident I had managed to organise everything food-wise.

Besides May and Annie's shop and the bakery, there was another small general grocery 'corner shop' quite near where I lived, run by an elderly Sark lady and her daughter. It was a typical village shop, with a bench inside the small room which was divided by a heavy polished wooden counter. It was so small I discovered the tradition was for just one customer to be attended to inside, while others sat outside on another bench until the shop was free. This was a bit of a chore in bad weather, but it was regarded as bad manners to crowd into the shop itself while someone was being served. I learned to check the number of waiting customers before deciding to call there.

One of the biggest attractions was that they sold home produced bacon, eggs and vegetables as well as locally made marmalade, jams and chutney, so I 'signed on' as soon as I could. I was not sure how I would be received as an English resident, but Hap and Sam were related somehow, and my suitability was guaranteed. Over time, as I treated more and more Sarkese I became totally accepted, and I was to thank these ladies for welcome help when deciding how much of any commodity I would need to feed my guests.

For its size Sark was well supplied with shops. Most of them were to be found in 'The Avenue;' a long lane at the top of the Harbour Hill. Approaching from that direction, there were two solid granite gate posts, and I was told these and the lane itself were once the access to the original Seigneurie or residence of the 'Ruler.' This building was now called the 'Manoir' and was divided into residential accommodation, mainly owned by an elderly lady related to the present Dame Sybil, and who eventually became a regular patient of mine.

Over the years the land bordering the Avenue had been divided into small freehold plots and now it had developed into the 'commercial area.' There was a butcher, small drapery, a cottage tearoom, a jeweller, the bakery, May's shop and a Post office cum stationers cum general hardware shop. This latter was called 'The Gallery' as it had been just that many years ago, built by the writer and artist Mervin Peak for his arty friends.

The butcher's shop was my next port of call when organising my menus. Much of the meat was local and I was delighted to discover I could get all my needs from Fred the butcher. I had been warned he was a 'character' and it was best to get on the right side on him as he had a hot temper, not averse to refusing to serve his customers if he took a dislike to them. So my first visit had me a little concerned. If this went wrong, I would have to get my meat from Guernsey, relying on the erratic boat service. The man himself had the appearance of the quintessential butcher, with rosy cheeks and bloodstained striped apron. I introduced myself and added I was opening Le Close des Camps as a guest house again and hoped he would be able to help me.

'You see, I've not done this before. I love cooking good food, and I've been told your meat is special and mostly local, which is what I want to give my guests.'

I had hit the right note, as Fred beamed and said he would be pleased to help me.

'I'll need to know what you want in advance, mind.'

'I've planned fourteen menus and I can tell you in advance; no problem...the only thing is...well I'm not sure how much I should order.'

'That's a'right; that's a'right: just tell me how many you are cooking for and I'll do the rest, Mrs Davies.' Over the years he was true to his word, although I learned to adjust numbers depending on the meat; for joints he tended to oversupply and for steak and kidney, I needed to add a few to the numbers.

The time came for the arrival of my first guests from Holland. Jeanne, Pieter and young Jos Vaasson were the perfect first guests. Jeanne was not much older than me, and we developed a rapport. I was impressed with their command of the English language, and I ruefully regretted we English made little effort to learn other languages as efficiently.

Jos adored Hugo, now all wagging tail and huge paws as they romped on the front lawn. Pieter was a reporter, and we could not have had better free publicity. When they returned home he wrote a delightful article about Sark and Le Clos des Camps, and for years we had people booking on the strength of Pieter's words.

When Ken was finally back on Sark, I felt our adventure could begin properly. On our frequent phone conversations I could detect an impatience in my usually phlegmatic husband to be able to leave his birthplace of

London and join me. I was not really convinced the few extra pounds of tax refund merited his decision to delay his moving fully to Le Close des Camps. I would have been too impatient to get started; but then our temperaments were so different. I just hoped we would cope, being together for twenty-four hours of the day. It was going to be vastly different from our life so far.

It was a late Easter and so the Island was at its best at the later part of April. The trees had unfurled their bright leaves, and every bank was thick with creamy primroses, pink and red campion and violets in clusters. On my return shopping trips, I had noticed the beauty of the cliffs, so rich with bright yellow gorse, sea thrift and bluebells; they looked like a large, designed garden. Memories of busy noisy London retreated to the back of my mind, and soon I was to be more fully occupied with nursing on the island.

Hap had been calling in occasionally for his 'wet' and I think he was keeping an eye on me, bless him, in his gruff way.

One day just before Easter on his visit, he was unusually quiet, and I asked him what the matter was. He had been munching on a piece of cake, which I was rather pleased to have baked successfully in the Rayburn.

'What is it, Hap? Is the cake that bad?'

'No it's OK for an English cook. Look, you said you want to do some nursing.' He took a huge bite. 'Well, it's my Annie. She's expecting her third as you know and still won't go to Guernsey to have it, eh?'

He licked the crumbs off his fingers and gave a small belch. 'S'cuse; she had the other two here; no problem. Well, will you go and see her about it?'

'Er, well, yes, but ... ,'

'Good, that's settled then.' He was gone before I could say anything more.

3/11

As Hap had been so kind to me, I felt I just had to call and see Annie again, but I was far from confident about assisting Dr King with a delivery in a basic home environment. While we had emergency midwifery instructions during the QIDN training and I had studied a few midwifery textbooks, I had not even seen a baby born at that time.

Annie had not been serving on my recent visits to the shop, and I was alarmed to see how large she had become when she invited me into the kitchen. It looked as if the baby was due any day.

'Your dad says you are still determined to have this baby here, Annie?'

'Like I told you Mrs Chris, I am not going to Guernsey; I'll deliver it myself if I have to.'

I had spoken to Dr King about Annie, and he had agreed he would attend the determined young woman, providing I was there to help, if I could not persuade her to go to the maternity hospital in Guernsey.

'But I haven't actually seen a baby born, let alone assisted.'

'You know how set everything up, and attend afterwards, though? If the pregnancy is straight forward, I don't see a problem.'

So, I reluctantly agreed with Annie.

'We first need to organise the birthing room.' I was taken to the house next to the shop where Sam, Annie and their two children, Jerry and Louise lived. It was a typical prefabricated bungalow consisting of a cosy dining kitchen with the inevitable Rayburn, three bedrooms, a small lounge, which seemed hardly used, and a bathroom.

'I'm going to have baby in Louise's room; she can bunk up with Gerry for a few days. Less trouble, eh?'

The room had a little cot and the single bed made up all ready.

'I've put a waterproof under the sheet, and there's a hot water bottle wrapped in a towel already and everything else we need, eh?' She indicated a neat pile of old clean towels and newspapers and showed me a drawer of tiny baby clothes.

'You are well organised, Annie.'

'Done it before, haven't I?'

I was liking this bright young woman with her 'no nonsense' attitude more and more. She never stopped working, even helping Hap and Sam in the farm occasionally when needed. She would have three young children under five to cope with, but they were a close family with five generations living on the Island, and I guessed they would all help.

'We had better sterilise some sani-pads, gauze and cotton wool balls. If you have an empty biscuit tin…?'

Annie hobbled to the shop and gave me a square tin with *"Huntley and Palmers' Family Circle"* on the paper cover so I pealed this off revealing the metal tin. After the inside was cleaned, I packed the dressings I thought we might need, along with some lengths of string to tie the chord and a pair of sharp scissors as Dr King had instructed me. I told Annie how to sterilise the tin and contents, and then all we had to do was wait.

A few days later the phone started to ring at two in the morning, and I suspected the baby was on the way. It was confirmed as soon as I heard Sam's voice; 'I'm on my way with the tractor, Mrs Chris.' I was thankful I had received permission from the constables to be collected by tractor for night calls. I decided to hitch my bike on the link box at the back as I had no idea how long it would be, and I guessed Sam would need the transport for the morning milking.

Dr King was there when I arrived and after examining Annie, nodded.

'Yes, it's on the way, but the head is not properly engaged yet; could be a while. Call me when the waters break,' and with that he left.

I was offered a cup of tea and Annie and I chatted for a while, but she was restless, wandering round the kitchen, stopping to grasp a chair back as a contraction hit her. After a while I realised these were far more often and when suddenly there was a flood of water as she groaned, I realised the birth was progressing more rapidly that the doctor had expected. I remembered reading a second or third birth could be very rapid and called to Sam, who was in the sitting room, to ring for the doctor, urgently.

'Come on Annie, time to go into the bedroom and lie down. I need to have a look what's happening.' What I saw when I examined Annie, galvanised me into action as I was sure it looked like the top of the baby's head all ready to be delivered. Just as I was opening the sterile tin and getting the linen ready for the doctor's arrival, Sam poked his head through the door.

'The doc's wife said he had to go out to an emergency...er what can I do?' I indicated the hot water bottle and asked him to fill it just as Annie started to grunt and exclaim, 'It's coming, its coming: I want to push Chris.' I remembered reading a baby should be born during controlled contractions and it could be delayed a little by the mother panting. I asked her to do this and then when she wanted to bear down again, I delivered the tiny head, which immediately shot out a jet of amniotic fluid from its little rosebud mouth. I knew I had to feel to make sure the chord was not round the baby's neck, thankfully finding nothing there. I wiped the little eyes with damp cotton wool, cleared the mouth and in the next contraction I delivered the upper shoulder. Smoothly then the lower shoulder slid out to be followed by the rest of a lovely little girl. As soon as the umbilical cord stopped throbbing, I tied it off and wrapped Sark's newest arrival in a warm towel as she yelled in indignation.

'Annie, you have a beautiful perfect little girl; well done.' It was then I realised this brave young woman had had no relief from the pain but had just got on with the job in hand.

With the birth successfully achieved, I was not sure about the afterbirth and what I was supposed to do. I knew the chord had to be cut and the afterbirth delivered, but thankfully I heard the doctor's voice, and he entered the room quickly.

'I am so sorry, Christine. I came as quickly as I could...but it looks as if you managed very well.'

'Not sure about the afterbirth, though...'

It only took a few minutes to tie the chord again, cut it and deliver the afterbirth. It was only then, as I carried the little mite to her mother, I realised Sam had not been told so I quickly went to the kitchen where he was anxiously waiting.

'Congratulations! You have a lovely healthy little daughter.'

'Is everything alright?'

'Mother and baby are doing well; do you want to go in?' I was not sure what the tradition was on the Island and hoped I had not upset anyone, but by the grin on Sam's face and smile on Annie's when I returned to the bedroom, there was no harm done.

Dr King was just packing up his bag, having given mother and baby a quick examination. He patted me on the shoulder in passing; 'Well done, nurse; well done.'

Little Valerie was making her presence known, so I helped Annie to give the new baby her first feed, while Sam returned to the kitchen. 'There'll be a glass of Sloe gin, when you're ready, Chris.' I noted with pleasure the dropping of the more formal address. Very few English residents were ever called by their Christian name by the Sarkese.

Little Valerie had fallen asleep, so I tucked her in the warmed cot while I washed Annie and made her comfortable. I had some idea a baby should be washed also but was not sure about this so asked Annie.

'That's alright Chris...can I call you that?...I'll see to my baby after a little sleep; you go and wet Valerie's head.'

Sitting in the warm kitchen, I took a tentative sip at the rich red liquid Sam had offered me. I did not normally like Gin, but this was smooth and fruity. I later learned Sloe Gin was a speciality in the Islands, made from the small bitter damson-like fruit of the blackthorn steeped in Gin and sugar and left to mature for months.

I also discovered it was potently alcoholic.

As the dawn was breaking, I cycled wearily but elated back home, realising I had just brought another being into the world. What I did not realise was that morning's work was as good as ten years' residency in establishing us on Sark.

3/12

For a week or so I continued to visit Annie and little Valerie, who thrived on the attention of her two siblings and the many members of her family. She became used to being handled, and as soon as her mother had recovered from the birth and was back serving in the shop, Valerie was usually there sleeping in her pram.

I had to admit Annie had been right in staying at home as it turned out, but much later when I took my midwifery training I was horrified to read of all the things that could have gone wrong.

Hap of course was delighted with his new grandchild, though did not say much in his visits for a 'wet.' Since Ken had arrived these were much less, and I was not sure if it was just because I was settled, or due to the fact he and Ken did not really get on. In any case I was glad to see him a couple of weeks after Valerie's birth. For once he was not very chatty, and even refused my cake. When I asked what the matter was, he hesitantly started; 'Annie and Sam have asked me to ask you, well that is; we would understand if...'

'Come on Hap, spit it out.'

'We wondered if you would agree to be one of little Valerie's godparents...we'd understand if you didn't want to, eh?'

For a moment I was speechless; it was almost unheard of for an English resident to be Godmother to a Sark child.

'Hap, I would be delighted.'

He grinned; 'That's alright then. How about that piece of cake, now, eh?'

In due time Ken and I attended the service in the Island's Anglican church, St Peter's. It looked as if half the Island's population attended, and I was very proud to hold little Valerie at the stone font. It was a very attractive church, built in the 1800s and I did not then realise how much I would be involved with it in the future. At the reception afterwards in the Island Hall, I met the rest of the extended family, and was fascinated to hear so much Sark Patois spoken. Many of the older generations spoke little English, and there were still several who had not been off the island for years. Try as I might I could never understand the strange language, traceable back to old Norman French, despite my working knowledge of modern-day French.

As if I had passed a test, more nursing cases came my way. A little while after Valerie's birth Dr King rang me one afternoon. We had only a couple of guests and I was organised for the evening meal.

'I wonder if you can help, Christine? An island lady living in Little Sark, Mrs Jacks has had a stroke and has a hemiplegia; I managed to get her in the ambulance by my surgery....' I could hear his sigh, 'but she just refuses to go to hospital in Guernsey in the Flying Christine where she really needs to be sent. Do you think you'd have a try as I must see another patient?'

The two-man emergency medical team was standing by with the patient in the ambulance, ready to be towed by tractor. The ruling that there were no cars allowed on the Island extended also to the ambulance and fire engine. The Sark ambulance was a converted caravan which had been fitted out with all the necessary first aid equipment; but it still had to be pulled by a tractor.

As I opened the door the patient glared at me.

'No! No! I not Guernsey: *I go home.*' Mrs Jacks mumbled from stiff lips. She was a woman of about sixty I guessed, of the stocky Island women's appearance: hair now untidily escaping from a bun of iron-grey hair and dressed in rough farming clothes. I had heard of the few families living on the small northern part of Sark, which was almost a separate island joined to 'Big Sark' by a three-hundred-foot-high isthmus called *'La Coupee.'* It was said they kept to themselves, seldom venturing into the bigger part of the Island.

I turned to Victor, the voluntary ambulance attendant. I had met him a few times and found his history fascinating. He had been a German medical orderly during the occupation of the Channel Islands and had been posted to Sark. He had met and fallen in love with a local lady and after the war, returned and married her. Now he had been the mainstay of the Sark Ambulance for many years. He had obviously been trying to persuade Mrs Jacks, without success. I suddenly had an idea.

'Does she have a husband, Victor? Yes? Well, where is he; can someone go and get him, please?' I thought it strange he was not there and should have been warned by Victor's elbow jabbing my ribs.

Mr Jacks soon arrived. He was surprisingly neat and well dressed, with a small moustache, so different from his wife's appearance. We had kept the ambulance door open, and our patient had agreed to lie propped up on the stretcher, so she could look out.

As soon as she saw her husband Mrs Jacks went very red in the face and I was concerned she was having another stroke. 'No: no: no.' She mumbled and gestured with her unaffected hand pointing at her husband. He in turn shrugged and asked in a disinterested voice, what the problem was. I was rather taken aback and explained she needed to go to Guernsey but refused. He just stood staring at the poor woman, shrugged and said, 'Not my problem, eh?' and walked off.

I reported to Dr King, telling him I had no success.

'Unfortunately, you can't make her go, so I guess you'll have to take her back home to Little Sark. I'll call in and see her when I can, but stay with her, will you?' I thought of the guests who would be wanting their evening meal so asked the Doctor to ring Ken. Most of it was ready and I knew he would be able to cope with just two guests.

We had to take Mrs Jacks home to Little Sark over the Coupee. I had been over it a few times by foot as cyclists were asked to dismount as it was steep and could be dangerous in strong winds. Only one tractor width, it had been fenced on each side and the road made substantial as recently as the end of the last war by German prisoners. Before that it had been rough with only a light rail. I had seen pictures of people crawling from one side to the other in gale force winds, in danger of being swept to the beach below. The journey in a swaying caravan over the high narrow causeway with sheer drops each side, made me feel like a second stretcher case, as I peered through the window, with memories of my sea trips between the islands.

Sight of the two-storey cottage did not cheer me as we drove up to Mrs Jack's farmhouse. The bedroom was up a steep flight of stairs. 'How on earth are we to get the patient up there?' I asked Victor.

The team had done this before.

Mrs Jacks was strapped into the stretcher and was hauled up headfirst. Just as we were about to lift her onto the bed, she mumbled something.

Bending down I asked her to repeat. 'Will go now; Guernsey!' I had been talking to the patient all the way. Whether it was that, or sheer bloody mindedness, she had suddenly decided that she *would* go over to the hospital in Guernsey after all.

Everything was done in reverse. We contacted the St John Headquarters in Guernsey; they sent the ambulance launch, Flying Christine 3, and we drove the patient to the Maseline harbour.

As we finally saw the ambulance launch off, I turned to Victor.

'Why was the husband so unhelpful and she looked mad at him, too. You would think he would be sympathetic.'

'Not really,' Victor grinned. 'I tried to warn you. They haven't lived together or spoken for years!'

From that day I decided to listen more to local gossip.

3/13

As the weeks and months went by, Ken and I settled into a routine. To my surprise I enjoyed being a guest house owner. My fear of having too much housework to do was not realised as there was little dust, our house being well removed from the unmade roads, and the air was so pure. Having no cars meant no petrol fumes; the only aromas wafting our way were from the many horses and carriages which passed by daily loaded with visitors.

Having only one bathroom and toilet combined did make some extra work, as we followed the Island tradition of supplying bowls and jugs of hot water to each room. The needs for relief during the night was catered for by an old-fashioned potty under each bed. After years of nursing, I was not squeamish about emptying them each morning.

One of the biggest problems Ken and I had to surmount was our relationship. Living and working together twenty-four hours a day was a far cry from the usual marriage. In London, we saw each other briefly in the morning as we rushed off to work. In the evening, I was often working, or Ken would be out with the badminton youth club or the scouts group he ran.

I discovered the fairy tales had it all wrong. It was impossible to live together happily ever after. Or maybe Prince Charming did not scatter coal all over the kitchen floor when he stoked the Rayburn or pull all the bedclothes off when he got up to the toilet in the freezing night. I bet the princess never had monthly problems or days when nothing went right. I was quite sure not many couples had to sleep in a storeroom when all the bedrooms were occupied, where a sudden movement sent a shower of toilet rolls or packets of cornflakes cascading over their heads. Nor were they woken in the night by the rattling water pump filling the tank, when a guest made a nocturnal visit to the bathroom.

But we survived and learned to laugh a little together.

Ken was pretty good at standing in when I was called on to visit a patient in the night, but that did not happen very often. Mostly I managed to fit my visits around my daily routine. The fact we had decided not to offer lunches meant as soon as we had cleared the breakfasts, and I had organised any preparation for the evening meal, I was free. It had been a point of discussion between us about lunches, but as I pointed out, most people went out for the whole day and would not want to come back. We did think about packed lunches, but Ken hit on the idea of a 'self-service shop,' which proved very popular. On a sideboard in the dining room we left packets of crisps, biscuits and small bars of chocolate for people to pay into an honesty box. On request I would make up a small bag of salad and cheese squares, and fresh fruit. As I gave a large breakfast and evening meal, that satisfied most people. Most guests were honest, but some did pocket bread and butter from the breakfast table. An innovation we had devised, from an abundance of toasters as wedding presents, was to give each table the chance to make their own toast so there was a good supply of fresh cut bread and pats of butter.

I gradually collected a few patients, either from the doctor or from phone calls. Most were to wash the elderly or cut their toenails; not in itself interesting nursing, but I become acquainted with some of the residents. Sometimes I was called on to lay out a departed elderly person, as there was no official undertaker on the Island.

Occasionally my nursing services were called upon by our guests.

3/14

Only having four rooms to let to guests posed a small problem. We encouraged families to visit but if there were children, parents expected a reduced rate, and it was not economic to give them a room too. We hit on the idea of 'family rooms' with bunk beds for the children and a double or two singles for the parents. We even bought a couple of cots for the very young ones. We were then quite happy to reduce the rates.

Very occasionally an adult family of four would be happy to share and take advantage of the reduction in cost. Such a family were the Jones' as we were fully booked otherwise. When I met the two couples, I was not too happy, as the in-laws looked quite elderly, but they all had been told about the bunk beds before booking so it was their choice.

'That's alright Mrs Davies; we often go Youth Hostelling and are used to this.' I was surprised the older couple took the bunk beds, but they seemed happy with the arrangement and enjoyed going out each day exploring our beautiful Island.

It was in their second week, when they announced at supper time they had all walked to Little Sark, had a cream tea at the Sablonnerie Hotel, and then climbed down the steep three hundred steps to the Grand Greve beach. This was something even I would have found a little strenuous.

That night we were awoken by a timid knock on our door. It was the young woman from this family; 'So sorry to disturb you, but Dad doesn't seem too well.'

Too much rich Sark Cream I thought, but followed while Ken grumbled and turned over in bed.

The snoring breathing, dribbling mouth and lack of responses from the elderly man, galvanised me into action. Even though he was on the top bunk, I managed to turn him on his side to stop him choking, asking his relatives to call Ken to ring urgently for the doctor.

Ken only had to crank the handle twice and told Mrs West the problem. Immediately she phoned the doctor, and after he visited and confirmed my suspicions, she put the emergency service into action. Within a quarter of an hour the Sark ambulance arrived, and the St John rescue launch started on its half hour journey from Guernsey. Victor and his driver were strong men and with the help of the patient's son and Ken, the whole bunk bed was lifted down and through the bedroom door. The Sark ambulance arrived at the Maseline harbour with the patient and his family, just as the launch from Guernsey rounded the headland. It was a well-practiced and perfected system, which had the patient in Hospital in Guernsey within an hour after the doctor's visit. I was pleased to hear our guest made a good recovery and they all came back the following year, but I insisted on separate rooms.

After our first year of taking summer guests, I was fortunate to be approached by the doctor to take a winter patient who had had a stroke. We still had a large loan to pay back to Ken's father, and we had no winter income.

'I've got an elderly lady in Little Sark,' he sounded unusually hesitant, 'she has had a stroke but pointedly refuses to go to Guernsey.' He continued, 'it has been twenty-four hours and she is no worse: trouble is, the son who is looking after her hasn't a clue.' He paused for a moment. 'I hear you are opening for the winter. She is not the easiest of customers, but could you take her in for a while?'

I had heard about Mrs Hill and her strong personality, but we badly needed the money, and she was 'not short of a bob or two' as my Dad would say. I agreed, and that afternoon my patient arrived: as did her dog. I was not happy about the yappy Jack Russell, but it was too late to change my mind. Hugo was easy going, and put up with the canine visitor and in the end they became good friends with Hugo teaching the smaller dog some manners.

I had nursed many patients after a stroke when I was in London, so this was no problem, but I realised Mrs Hill was not going to be easy. I welcomed her with a cup of tea and a piece of homemade cake...I had mastered the Monstrosity by then...and started as I meant to continue. I knew too much softness was no help in the healing process.

'Right, Mrs Hill,' I said firmly as soon as she was finished, 'time to get up for a sit in the chair.' My patient mumbled something. 'Sorry didn't catch that. Try just one word.' I certainly heard the resounding '*No*' that time.

I looked the elderly woman in the eye as she glared at me and I folded my arms.

'Look, I could just let you lie there all day, getting bedsores and deteriorating to a zombie, or we can work together on this.' I wondered if I had gone too far, but saw a small glint in Mrs Hill's eye, before she turned her head away.

Pulling a chair to the bedside, I tried a different tack. 'I hear you have had an interesting life, and I would love to hear all about it.' I saw a glint of humour in her bright blue eyes, and I knew the healing process had begun.

Daily my patient made progress. Even the dog and I had an armed truce when he learned who fed him. Gradually my patient's speech returned, and I soon had her telling me stories of her exciting life of world travel and of her time as a cook in a Canadian Lumber Camp. I particularly delighted in one of her favourite sayings, when we had been chatting for a long time. 'My dear Chris, we really have been hung up by the tongue today!'

From passive exercises to her weakened arm and leg, to tentative walks round her room, to exercises outside when the weather permitted, gradually Mrs Hill made an excellent recovery. After four weeks, she left with only a slight limp, but by the time she left, my thoughts of possibly opening an old people's home were banished forever. I had found the combination of nursing and cooking breakfast, lunch, supper, and supplying innumerable snacks and cups of tea, exhausting, but I did agree to take another patient the following winter.

Mrs Bentley had also had a stroke but was more ambulant and just wanted a few weeks of care and 'cosseting' as the doctor put it. It did not mean so much work, and the nursing was minimal. She was a true lady and was obviously used to servants but did not treat me as one. Always immaculately dressed this slim, white-haired guest was appreciative of all I did for her.

Which of course made me want to do more.

I was still able to continue helping Ken with outside repair work. All the fifty-two small windows in the conservatory had lost their putty, and I thought I would like to try my hand at its replacement. I had read that if *Pollifiller* was mixed with half water and half gloss paint it worked like putty, so I donned my grubbiest clothes and mixed a large dish-full.

It was a rare winter sunny, wind-free day; the birds had started to sing and I thought I could smell the grass growing. I looked over at the front lawn, thinking it would soon need cutting. And to my horror, I saw 'La Dame's' electric invalid chair stop by our gate.

She got out and started to walk across the lawn using her stick to support her arthritic hip. I rushed over, putty and pallet knife in hand.

'It's alright, Mrs Davies. I haven't come to see you. I can see you are busy.' I could see a twitch of humour on her lips. 'I have come to see my friend Beatrice. Maybe we could have a cup of tea and a slice of your famous cake, when you have finished.' I abandoned the rock-hard batch of putty and changed to cleaner clothes.

After all, it was not every day that your 'Head of State' came to tea.

3/15

We soon decided to use the remainder of our two fields which were not planted with vegetables, to start a smallholding. Our first acquisition was two hives of bees. These came from an elderly man whom I attended for a while, but then he decided to move to Guernsey. I had told him Ken was interested in beekeeping but neither of us knew anything about the subject, and as far as I was concerned it was the only part of our planned self-sustenance I could not face. I had been stung once as a child and the reaction was painful and long lasting. It left me with a fear which bees were able to sense and made them aggressive in my presence, but I was intrigued with the stories Mr Smith told me while I helped him wash, shave and dress.

'Did you know,' he would say, 'when a worker has found a good source of pollen and nectar, she will show the others where it is?' He smiled at me. 'Clever little things! She will do a dance on the alighting board of the hive to show them the location.'

'You said 'she', are they all female?'

'The workers, yes. The drones are the male; only use is to breed with the Queen on her maiden flight. Then a lot of them are bumped off!' He wheezed in laughter. 'Should happen to all of us useless males.'

'No, don't say that. I shall miss you. You've made me see how amazing bees are. I've always been a bit scared of them. Ken wants to have a few hives, and I can see why.'

'I've had an idea; how would you and your hubby like to take a couple of my hives?'

'I couldn't do that: I am sure you could sell them.'

'What say you take them as exchange, instead of giving me a bill? That should keep you both happy. 'Nuff said; decision made.' He would not change his mind and that was how we started in the beekeeping business.

Our next enterprise was to acquire a few hens. Obtaining sufficient fresh supplies for our guests was expensive and unreliable as the cargo delivery depended so much on the weather. So we bought a henhouse on wheels and started with just twenty four young pullets. As with the bees, we bought books on poultry rearing, for we knew little about either. Gradually news travelled round the Island that we had fresh eggs, and so we eventually ended up with about two hundred hens in 'fold units' which were moved around daily. The hens were released late in the afternoon to free range, as laying was mostly done in the morning.

Our next acquisition was a couple of goats, from the Island of Guernsey. We knew nothing about these animals either, but Sam came to our rescue and showed us all we needed to know.

Finally we bought a donkey, Pedro, to pull a cart to deliver our growing produce and help with the shopping.

As if I was not busy enough with the animals, guest house and occasional nursing patients I was hankering to start a family. Ken was a little reluctant, although we had discussed this before we were married, agreeing it would be nice to have two children.

'Don't you think you have enough to do, Chris?'

To which I replied in all innocence, 'It'll be just like another animal, won't it?'

How wrong can you be?

It was not long before I fell pregnant, but I nearly lost the baby before I knew I was expecting as I had a painful accident.

I was trampled by one of Jim's horses.

One day Ken had gone for a walk with Hugo, and I was in the kitchen attending to some letters when I heard our donkey making a terrible din in the field behind the house. Dropping everything I rushed out to see our poor little animal racing round and round on his chain, trying to avoid the teeth of a huge white horse. I recognised Prince, one of our carter Jim's horses. They were always escaping from his badly fenced fields. Having believed for years donkeys and horses were inseparable and natural companions, I had discovered some horses simply hated donkeys. This brute was obviously one of them.

Giving no thought to my safety, as I was sure the horse would back off, I rushed out to unclip Pedro and lead him to the stable. I did not know that Prince also hated women.

I felt a hard push in the middle of my back and fell face down on the grass, the horse rearing above me, snorting through his flared nostrils.

Twice I felt a searing, burning pain in my left buttock and thought I had been bitten, and two local boys, taking a short cut through the next field saw it all. They told me afterwards a hoof had landed close to my spine; further over and it would probably have snapped like a twig. I lay there for an unbelieving moment, then rolled over and over to escape the huge rearing hooves. Receiving a glancing blow on a shoulder and hip, I scrambled up and staggered to the house, shaking with shock. The two lads raced to Ken who was just returning and told him what had happened. As he dashed into the house to see me, the boys chased the horse out of our field. It was then the tears started, but I could only think of poor Pedro, and insisted he be stabled first before I allowed Ken to phone the doctor.

I went to bed and found I was bleeding. I thought the shock had brought on a period; I realised much later it must have been a threatened miscarriage.

The following guest house season was a busy one, and I was not able to rest as much as I should have done. Whether it was this or the shock of the accident, my little son Roy was born a month prematurely as I had developed toxaemia.

He was a fretful infant, and I found my earlier blithe comments about a baby being no more trouble than another animal was totally inaccurate. The pressure was too much for me and I nearly had a breakdown.

We had been running our business for seven years, with no breaks for a holiday and one day when Roy was nearly three years old, Ken returned from a trip to Guernsey dropping two library books on the table. There were magical pictures of lakes and mountains on the cover.

'I was just thinking, Roy is getting nearly to three and it won't be long before he goes to school.' He gave me a frank look, 'I think this life is getting you down a bit; I could do with a change for a year or two, as well.

I looked at the front of the first book. 'New Zealand!' I exclaimed.

'Well, if we want to have a look at it, we'd better do it before Roy's five.'

I looked at the two men in my life and felt the familiar surge of excitement returning.

'Why not?' I said.

So that was how I left our Island paradise for a while, to tour New Zealand with Ken and Roy, and finally move there in 1976; but I was not finished with the magical Island.

****

Sadly, Ken and I went our separate ways in 1984 and I was to return to Sark with the love of my life, Peter to live a totally different lifestyle, and to take up again my post as Island Nurse.

****

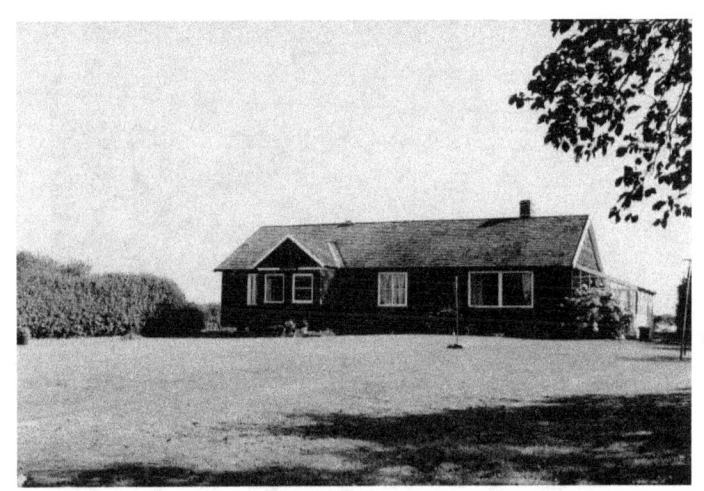

Le Clos des Camps

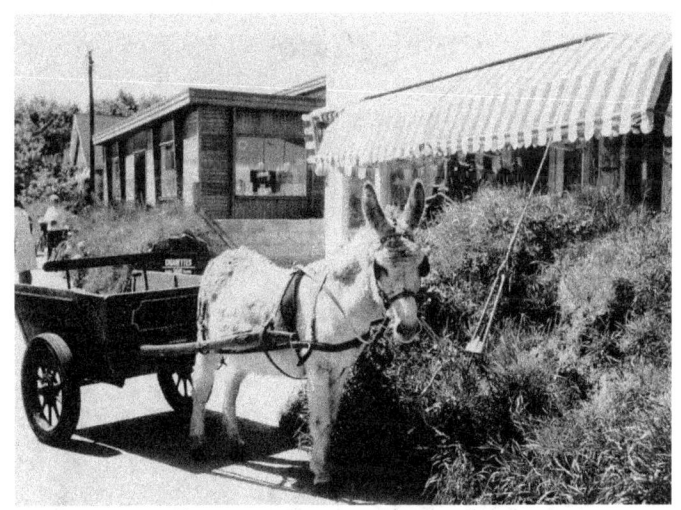

Shopping Sark-style

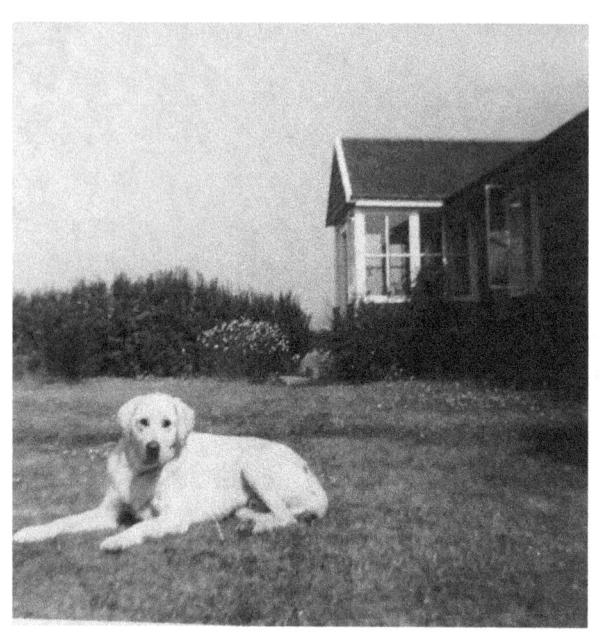

Hugo

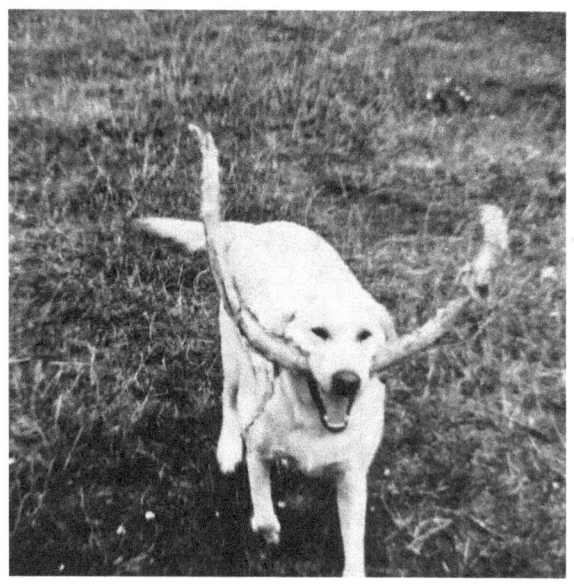

3/16

Marjorie and Peter Curtis arrived on Sark a couple of years after we did and ran a very successful guest house and tea garden. As was the habit among guest house owners, we often shared bookings of guests if we could not accommodate them, particularly the occasional party who arrived on the Island without booking; not a very good idea. In high season every bed was normally booked well in advance.

A friendship grew between us, and often Peter would help us out with the smallholding if we needed to be away for a night or two to go to Guernsey. In the winter we four joined the badminton club, and sometimes attended to local dance at one of the Island's pubs.

While Marjorie was quiet and a little introverted, like Ken, Peter and I were more fun loving and we often danced together, leaving our spouses to sit and observe. Peter was the type to dominate a dance floor with his well-meaning exuberance. I found his zest for life refreshing and laughter was never far away when he was around. Over the years he became a good friend and we talked together about anything and everything.

When Ken, Roy and I moved to New Zealand, Peter and I wrote to each other, and he was very interested in that country. I think if he had not needed to help finance his three children through tertiary education, and if Marjorie had been keener, he might have tried his luck there. He was a well-educated, university man from a privileged background and I think Ken had a slight feeling of inferiority, not having had his opportunity.

They were not close friends.

In our letters to each other over the years we got to know each other very well, and gradually each confided to the other our unhappiness in our marriages. For me it was a relief to unburden myself, but I felt a little self-critical at not being content with my lot. Ken and I had fallen into a rut, but I knew after many years of marriage that often happened. I felt my problem was my lack of maturity when I married. With my sheltered home life and then as a student nurse, I had little experience of relationships. I had not had a serious boyfriend before I met Ken at the age of eighteen. As a mature man of twenty-seven, he was the man he was going to be, while my character was yet unformed. My responsibilities as a nurse and the many other activities had changed me, sadly away from the person Ken thought I was. We had a few uncomfortable discussions of where we were going in our marriage and had thought of a trial separation when Roy was older.

In 1981 I had a windfall of a small legacy from a relative I had not known existed and thought it would be a good idea for Roy, then thirteen years old, to visit his grandparents in England. I tried to persuade Ken to come with us, but he felt he could not leave the small beekeeping business he had started.

'Come on, Ken, you can spend some of that "Rainy day fund," you talk about.' I did not know what his income was: I had never known and had accepted that as this was how it had been in my own family. I had agreed we would mostly live off my reasonably high salary as a rural district nurse, with a house and car included, but I did not see why Ken could not spend a little of his money on a fare over to see his mother, at least.

Ken was adamant: maybe he welcomed some time on his own, but whatever the reason, Roy and I journeyed alone via Los Angelis and Disneyland to England. We first visited my parents in Yorkshire and then I left Roy with his Nana to be spoiled rotten in London, while I journeyed back to Sark.

I had not been there for five years and knew a few of the changes from Peter's letters, but basically it was still the same. I also knew the situation between Peter and Marjorie had deteriorated, and he had moved out of the old cottage he and Marjorie had bought a few years ago, into a tiny second cottage in the grounds.

Peter was waiting at the Maseline harbour as I arrived, and I was quite unprepared for the jump in my heart when I saw his tall figure on the quay. The hug he gave me nearly drove the breath from me, and the physical contact stirred forgotten feelings I had long pushed away. As I looked at his familiar face; not handsome but 'lived in' and full of character, I noticed a cut where he had shaved; his hair needing a trim and a button was missing on his shirt, and my heart went out to my dear friend; and stayed there. It only needed his intense gaze and his voice saying 'Chrissie, Chrissie; welcome back to Sark,' to make me realise I was deeply in love with my special friend.

In unaccustomed silence we walked to his Guest House where he had arranged for me to stay. He and Marjorie still ran the successful business, helped by two seasonal staff, and his two daughters and son when home from their education. I had always got on with Marjorie although we were not close friends as we had little in common, so I politely accepted the coffee and cake she offered, longing to be alone with Peter.

At last we were able to escape for a walk, and it was on the wild windblown Eperquerie common, sitting on the old wooden seat, we were at last able to declare our love for each other. Taking my hands Peter talked about a possible future together.

'Chrissie, I know we will have to wait till Roy and my three leave their education, but I am determined one day we must be together...in a cottage somewhere...or anywhere. What do you say?'

It all seemed so new to me and an impossible dream, but I went along with it for the short time we had together but knowing I would be seeing Peter again before very long. He told me an uncle who was interested in the family's genealogy had discovered distant relatives in New Zealand.

'He traced back to a secretary of Bishop Selwyn, the first Anglican Bishop of New Zealand and our relatives are now settled in Hawks Bay on land which was offered to them.'

He grabbed my hands. 'So, we will be coming out next year to visit my New Zealand relatives and we can meet up again. I want you to seriously think about us.'

The rest of our holiday went in a whirl, and I was soon back in New Zealand wondering how I was going to survive until I saw Peter again. Ken and I had agreed on single beds some years previously. I moved into the spare room, and we continued our parallel lives hoping not to affect our son Roy too much, but he must have known things were not happy at home.

The time came for Peter and Marjorie to arrive at Auckland Airport and Roy and I drove to meet them. Ken said he was too busy to come and anyway, as he pointed out, there would not be enough room in my small car. He generously offered to move out of the main bedroom, and sleep in an old caravan we kept in our large garden for the week Marjorie and Peter were to stay with us.

It was a strange week. Peter and I were longing to be together alone, and Marjorie was showing signs of the stress she felt in having to spend time with her estranged husband. It was almost a relief when they set off in a hired car to visit their relatives in Hawkes Bay. They were to spend the last few days of their visit with us, and I was determined to try and have Peter to myself for a short while. We did manage a few walks and it was wonderful to discover we still had a strong love for each other and renewed our vows one day to be together.

The final day of departure arrived, and Roy and I took Marjorie and Peter back to the airport. As Roy and I stood watching the plane depart I could contain myself no longer and burst into tears. That lovely son of mine...just a teenager...took hold of my arm and steered me to the cafeteria.

'I know Mum, I'm not blind. I could see you and Peter have something, er, special. You mustn't worry about me. I shall go to Uni and you must do what you need to do.'

He took a swig of his chocolate milk shake, 'I could hear you crying in your room and I know dad's not happy...'
Out of the mouths of babes....

3/17

Three more years rolled by, and the letters between Peter and me became more intimate, but we each carried on our lives until I received unsettling news from my mother early in 1984. My father's Parkinson's disease had deteriorated and now he had mild dementia as a complication.

I realised I needed to visit my parents before too long.

I could also see Peter again, and now Roy was approaching his sixteenth birthday maybe Peter and I could look at a future together. Roy now had a special girlfriend from his class in school and he was planning to go to university: he seemed to have a stable future. Ken was very much involved with the scouts and the Baden Powel League, spending time away from home at weekends and evenings. I had been seriously thinking of moving to a small flat offered to me by some friends, and discussed it with Ken, but decided to delay until I returned from my trip to UK.

I was met at the airport by Peter, and it was as if we had never been apart. Any doubt I might have had of my feelings for him was dispelled, as we talked while he drove to a small cottage he had booked in the Lake District. Here we spent a few wonderful days together before I caught the train to Yorkshire, planning to meet up with Peter again in Gloucestershire after a couple of weeks with my parents. I was relieved to discover my father was not as incapacitated as I had expected and was pleased I had made the trip when I did. I knew his prognosis was not good.

Peter's two daughters were both married and lived in Gloucestershire, and I had several friends in the area, so it was a suitable place for our second holiday together. I wanted to visit Allie who was a farmer in the area near a delightful village called Northleach. We had been at secondary school together and I had spent many happy days with her at her father's farm during weekends and holidays. I had always been a bit of a 'tomboy' and loved driving the old grey "Ferguson" tractors and working in the fields. She was a lively ebullient young woman and I thought she and Peter would get on well; which they did when we called at her picturesque old Cotswold stone farmhouse.

While Peter went to look at the old fourteenth century church oposite, Allie and I caught up with our news over a cup of coffee and cake.

'Oh, Chrissie; your Peter is right for you. I often wondered why you married Ken.'

'Well, it seemed like a good idea at the time.'

'What are you going to do? You mustn't let him get away.'

I was almost in tears; feeling pulled this way and that.

'I just don't know.'

I did not realise at that time I would be spending some months with Allie and her husband in her lovely home.

All too soon it was time for Peter to drive me back to Heathrow airport. After my time with Peter, I could not face the atmosphere at home and felt the best plan was for me to accept the offer of a friend's flat near the district nursing office, temporarily. I had written to Ken to tell him of my decision.

Having booked in at reception and weighed in my suitcase, I decided to phone my mother.

I was in for a shock.

'Oh, Chrissie; I've had a letter from Ken, and he said he knew you would phone me...' I could hear the tears in her voice as she read; *"Tell Chris if she does not come back and live as before, she need not come back at all."*

There was a ringing in my ears and my heart was pounding. 'Just a minute, Momma, read that again. I don't understand. Ken and I had agreed I was coming back to New Zealand to live separately and try and sort things out. We can't go on as things are.' She read the whole letter and it seemed Ken had not come to terms with what I had understood was a joint decision. I knew he was concerned about the financial side, but I had assured him on that count.

The ringing had stopped, and I felt I was floating. I could not hear the airport noises nor see the people hurrying past the phone kiosk. There was an artificial stillness in me, and I heard a voice...my voice...saying calmly. 'Well, I'm just not going back to New Zealand just yet then: I must sort myself somehow. I will contact you when I know what I am doing: must go: don't worry.' I hung up and turned to Peter who had been waiting patiently. He stretched out his hand and gripped my arm. 'Are you OK? You're as white as a sheet!'

'I'm fine thanks.' The calm was still with me, and I felt as light as a feather. 'I'm not going back.'

'What?'

'I will never sort myself out if I go back to New Zealand just now. For all his words, Ken will not accept we are finished if I am there.'

'What about Roy?'

'He'll be O.K. I'll have to go back when I am sorted. He'll be off to university soon: he is nearly seventeen.' I had my first pain of indecision. My beloved son: how would I tell him his mother was leaving the family?

'It's not for ever:' but as I said it, I knew that I was changing all our lives irrevocably.

Peter's practical voice brought me back to reality.

'We'd better go to the airline desk and see if we can get your suitcase back.'

I was beginning to shake with shock at the enormity of what I had decided to do. Yet in my heart was a deep relief at last I was able to take some action. There had been too many years of living parallel lives with little warmth on either side of our marriage.

The airline staff were most sympathetic. Peter explained to them I had to cancel my flight due to an emergency. I suppose they could see from my face that I was very upset.

'You're lucky Mrs Davies: your case has not gone out to the plane yet. We can open your return ticket. It will be valid for a year, but you may have to pay a little more if the fares go up.' I nodded, hardly able to think beyond the relief of not having to go back just yet, and to be able to spend more time with my Peter.

We sat in the cafeteria at the Airport, trying to make plans.

'What will you do: where will you go? Will you go to Yorkshire to stay with your parents?'

Gradually the numbness left me. I had to think.

'No: Ally said I could stay with her in the farmhouse. She did say I should stay longer and sort myself.' Peter looked as stunned as I felt, but again his common sense prevailed. He looked at his watch and said he would phone his elder daughter Lyn in Gloucester.

'I was going to stay with her for a few days before going back to Sark: I'll give her a ring and tell her a little of what has happened...' I opened my mouth to comment but Peter continued... 'no, I won't say much, just that you have had to stay on longer. She knows about us, you know.'

I felt my face turning red. 'I am not sure there is an 'us' yet. I need to find myself first.'

He took my hands in his. 'I think we need to be together; but I agree you must have some time on your own, but don't take too long to make up your mind.' With that he pushed my bag towards the exit and the hired car, and I walked beside him.

Lyn and her husband made us welcome, but they had no spare bedroom. The two children agreed to share and I had one room while Peter slept downstairs on a sofa bed.

'And no pussy-footing up and down the stairs in the night!' She said with a twinkle in her eye. I managed to get back to my bed just before the family stirred in the morning.

3/18

The next few days were best forgotten. I had to make the dreaded phone call to Roy and of course to Ken. They both took it quietly, and Roy showed a maturity beyond his years.

'I knew you were unhappy Mum. I could hear you crying sometimes; and when you moved to the spare room, well I knew there was something wrong.'

'Will you be O.K?'

'I was going to tell you about my girlfriend when you came back. She is in my class at school; in fact, we have been dating for a year or more...'

'Roy that's wonderful!' I had been concerned when my son had shown no signs of seriously going out with girls, even though he had mentioned a friendship with someone. I even had a thought that he may prefer his own sex.

'There's just one thing, Mum, she's in a wheelchair. She has spina-bifida.'

'Well, that's O.K. isn't it? Is she, er, alright?'

'Of course. She's one of the brightest in the class.'

'That's good. I'm glad for you. I think I'd better be going. I'll write when I have somewhere to stay.'

'Mum...?'

'Yes?'

'Don't worry. Will you be O.K?'

I choked back my tears. How I was going to miss my only child.

'I'll be O.K. I have Peter.'

I rang off and took a deep breath. The first hurdle was over: now I had to find somewhere to live and then get a job.

The day after my dramatic decision, Peter and I visited Ally again. She did not seem surprised as we rolled up to the old Cotswold stone farmhouse in our hired car, and as she opened the solid oak door, a clarion of bells rang out from the square church tower. We stood there grinning at each other, speech being impossible, as the joyful music rang and then Ally gave me a big hug.

'Well, I see you have taken my advice, Chrissie.' She gave Peter a kiss on his cheek and pulled us into the warm kitchen, heated by an 'Aga' stove. Over steaming cups of coffee and another piece of home-made cake I asked if her offer still stood of a room for a few weeks.

'Of course! When do you want to move in?'

I glanced at Peter and smiled, 'Er, Tomorrow?'

Everything was moving so rapidly I felt as if I was in a different world. I should have been arriving in New Zealand, and here I was following Allie up several flights of creaking stairs and along a narrow corridor right at the top of the house. She pushed open a door and we followed her into a bedroom which was going to be my home for rather longer than I had expected.

A huge bed dominated, with basic furniture wedged in where it would fit. There was a tiny wardrobe but as I only had one suitcase of clothes, it would be enough. The small window which nestled deep into the stone wall looked directly at the church and churchyard.

'How often does the church clock strike?'

'Every third hour: through the night as well.' Ally's grin did nothing to relieve me.

After a while, I became so used to the bells I hardly heard them. The only problem was, when someone phoned on the third hour it was impossible to talk for several minutes. The farmhouse had a grandfather, a grandmother and a granddaughter clock which were tuned to strike one after the other, following the church clock. Peter and I soon learned to avoid phoning one another at those times in the ensuing months.

Thoughtfully we wandered round the picturesque village. I did not take in very much of it at that time, though later was to fall in love with its pretty Cotswold stone cottages, gardens bursting with Spring flowers and the majestic Church, almost as large as a cathedral.

After a sandwich and cup of tea in a small tea shop we made our way back to Lyn's house in Gloucester, discussing my plans for the immediate future.

'You must have a car, Chrissie. I must go back to Sark, and you'll need to get about. Will you try to get a job?'

'It depends how long I stay. I will go to the local bank and open an account and transfer my money. I have my salary paid into a joint account, and there should be a few thousand to see me by.'

I was in for a shock.

I had no trouble opening an account, but when I asked to transfer what I needed, I was told there were only a few dollars there.

'I can't understand it...'

'Well, as a joint account with your husband, it looks as if he has withdrawn most of it. I am sorry Mrs Davies.'

Not as sorry as I was; and furious.

That night I rang Ken, catching him just before he left for work. 'Well, what did you expect Roy and me to live off Chris? You haven't thought this through, have you? You should have heard your son crying last night!'

If I had not been so furious, that would have upset me although later I discovered this was not strictly true.

'What about my car I was buying. The monthly payments come out of that account.'

There was silence for a moment, then Ken replied. 'I'll take that on for now. We can sort this out when you return.'

It was then I realised Ken had not totally accepted our separation as inevitable, but I rang off in frustration as I could not face any more confrontation. I was now destitute with just a suitcase of clothes and no job. I contacted my district nursing department in New Zealand, saying I had decided to stay on in England for an indeterminate time. Resigning, I apologised for any inconvenience, but they were very understanding, saying they would send a reference in the mail. Until it arrived I was not sure if I would be employed without one, but I could not wait for the post which may take a couple of weeks.

Peter had to return to Sark, but before he did, we searched for a suitable small car for me. We settled on an old Fiat Strada, battered but game. 'You can pay me back some time,' he said as the dear man handed me a sizeable cheque to keep me going until I was earning again.

Cheltenham, near Gloucester, is a popular town for wealthy retirees. The level terrain, many shops and pretty public gardens meant a fair number of retirement nursing homes had opened there. I spent a few days plodding from one to the other, hoping someone would accept me without a reference. As the holiday season was approaching, there were several places looking for relief staff. One small rest home accepted me, after asking about my experience, and with the understanding I should give them my reference as soon as it arrived from New Zealand.

'Can you work shifts, and some nights Mrs Davies?'

Yes, I could: I had nothing much else to do and knew few people in the area so I was not anticipating a social life.

It was agreed I could have an occasional weekend off as I was longing to spend some time with Peter again as he planned to come over as often as he could.

I entered a strange half-life.

As I spent time with Peter it became more and more difficult to think of a life without him even for a year or two. When he was not with me I could still feel his presence: when he phoned I would dash to answer, breathless as a teenager with her first love.

Ally was a great friend in need, absorbing me into her life effortlessly. I was interested in her herd of prize sheep and on one occasion I went with her to a local show in a neighbouring town.

'I'm a bit worried about the big ram. He's a randy old devil and if there are any ewes on heat, he'll be hard to handle.'

While I was a district nurse in New Zealand I had become interested in complementary medicine and particularly homeopathy. I had used Bach Flower Rescue Remedy sometimes in stressful circumstances and remembered being told it was effective in calming animals.

'Well, it won't do any harm.' Ally was obviously not convinced, until she admitted on the way home she had never seen the ram behave so well. 'What was that stuff called, Chrissie? I'll get a bottle full!'

It was one small thing I could do to repay her kindness.

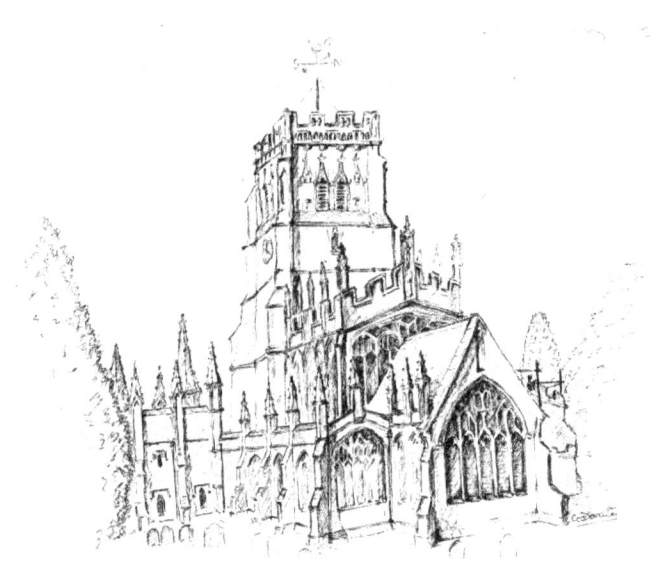

Nothleach Church

3/19

I had forgotten how bewitching early summer could be in England, especially in the rural Cotswolds. The fragrance in the air was intoxicating: a mingling of wildflowers, blossoms and lush growing greenery. The dawn was so early it seemed the sun had hardly set before the birds awoke to announce the new day with a joyful chorus. Wood pigeons cooed gently as a background to the trill of blackbird and thrush, with the strident cuckoo shouting his defiance above them all.

I had not realised how I had missed it all in the brasher, sub-tropical vibrancy of New Zealand. Now it acted as a balm to my tumbling emotions. I allowed myself to slip into my new life, avoiding making a decision about my future. It was enough to drive the old car to work along a country road: to park under the lush green trees and spend the day tending to my elderly patients. The work was not arduous, mainly looking after the twenty elderly people: washing or bathing them; dressing and handing out their medication. Some had had interesting experiences, and to listen to their stories took my mind off the strange life I was leading.

Back at the farmhouse I often cooked the evening meal for Ally and her husband. I enjoyed the luxury of using an Aga and learned how to stack a dishwasher, a novelty for me.

We would sometimes sit outside with a glass of wine as the days got warmer. Over the constant sound of cooing doves, I would have one ear listening for the frequent phone calls from Peter: my heart skipping a beat when I heard his familiar voice.

I realised I would have to decide soon. Ken was beginning to talk of separation: Roy was studying for exams, and although he was missing me, accepted the situation. I convinced myself, if I returned to New Zealand it would aggravate things again.

Peter came over to visit me frequently and I travelled over to Guernsey one weekend but did not venture over to Sark, but we discussed it one weekend. I had been in Northleach for a couple of months by then and Ken and I had been communicating by airmail. His letters often upset me so much I had to sit on the toilet to read them. I realised he had not really taken our situation seriously, and it had been a shock for him. He blamed Peter, but I knew sooner or later we would have had to move away from each other. The tension some of the time was hard to bear and I started to have migraine headaches, which had not ever plagued me before.

Roy and I spoke regularly on the phone, and he seemed happy enough, studying for final school exams and applying for university. His friendship with his girlfriend seemed very serious, and he was even talking of marriage in a few years. I was glad for him and her support but I longed to see him again.

'You know, Roy, they opened my air ticket and so we could put money towards a trip over in your summer holidays.'

'Won't it be cold though; it will be winter.'

'Switzerland would be OK wouldn't it?'

'Wow. Do you mean ski-ing?'

'Why not? Maybe your Uncle David will join us from Holland. He's an expert.'

We started to plan for this holiday, but in the meantime I had to decide about our property in Sark. We had sold a ten-year lease on our guest house business, and there were still eighteen months to run, but I needed somewhere to live if I was to stay on the Island.

Peter and I discussed this.

'I think I should visit Sark and talk to the tenants.'

'Yes, Chrissie, I think it is time for you to come back to Sark. I want you to come and live with me, but I can't offer you marriage, you know that.'

Many of the laws of this strange little Island were feudal. Some of the constitution had been brought up to date, and the system worked well but there were still some peculiarities. There was no mechanism in place to divorce a couple who both lived on the Island. One of them would have to leave the Island for a year and a day. If they did that, then they may possibly run into some residential problems on their return.

'What about Marjorie and your son, David?'

'Marjorie says you are welcome to me. She says you have always been her friend.' Peter said this with a wry expression.

'It is so bizarre. It all seems so unreal.' I was far from happy about living 'out of wedlock' but there was no alternative if we wanted to be together.

'It is very real, Chris. If you feel you can't face the gossip...and you know there will be some, maybe we should get a little cottage somewhere else.'

'I couldn't do that to you. You love the Island and the life there and your son David has just returned from Agricultural College. Didn't you say he had managed to get a lease on 'La Ville Farm?'

'Yes, well I was hoping to give him a bit of a hand in the renovations, but...'

'I love Sark too. No;' I made one of my snap decisions, 'I shall come back for a trial period. At least if they are gossiping about me they will give someone else a rest!'

I returned to Sark.

I first needed to see the couple with three small boys who had leased 'Le Clos des Camps' to see if they would sell the remainder of the lease back to me. My reception was not very friendly, and I was surprised. Despite a higher offer when we had advertised the business to lease, we had chosen them as being Channel Islanders. We felt they would be more at home with island life.

'You never answered our letter when we wrote to say we wanted to buy the place.' They said when I visited them.

I knew nothing of this and realised Ken had never discussed it with me, but the young couple did not believe me. I think they never forgave me, as they were not very friendly for the whole time I knew them. Despite their antagonism, as they were planning to build their own house, eventually they agreed to let me buy back the remaining part of the lease.

Now I had somewhere for Peter and me to live eventually.

We realised there was work to be done on Clos des Camps before we could move in, and to my surprise Marjorie came to the rescue. It as a bizarre situation. Although Peter had said his wife had declared that she did not want to live with him anymore, I could not really believe she would be so welcoming. We spent a few weeks in his guest house, and then Marjorie offered the small cottage in her grounds. Eventually we became an odd trio, often going out together to public functions and Peter gained a certain notoriety with his 'two wives.'

Marjorie's cottage was just a couple of fields away from Close des Camps so we spent as much time as we could looking over the old bungalow. What we saw was depressing.

'Just look at this.' Peter pushed open a window and it swung out on rusted hinges, nearly falling into the flower bed below. 'And there are leaks in two of the bedrooms. Is this the same roof as when the house was built in 1946?'

I assumed it was. The old cedar 'Colt' house had been built just after the war, not long after the German occupying force had been removed when the Island had been liberated. Apart from the new porch, little had been done besides repainting.

'It will need new windows and a roof, and I wouldn't be surprised if rain hadn't leaked from the window frames to the studs underneath.' Peter shook his head. 'Be better to knock it down and start again.'

'Well, it's not all mine yet anyway. Ken still owns half.'

Ken and I were reaching an agreement about our separation. He seemed much happier since Peter had offered to give a quarterly financial settlement to help Roy in his schooling and expenses. Peter's only stipulation was Roy was to give a breakdown of how the money was spent, which he was happy to do.

We came to an agreement that Ken would relinquish his half of Clos des Camps and I would sign over my half of the property we had in New Zealand. The value was not equal so I also had to give Ken a substantial cash payment. I was able to do that as Peter had purchased a half of Clos des Camps. Peter and I would then jointly own the property, but it was not a simple procedure under Sark law. Ken and I had first to sell it to a third party and then Peter and I had to buy it back.

At last the legal details were sorted and we could plan for the future. The problem was where to live while we re-built Clos des Camps The cottage we were in was only two rooms and a tiny bathroom.

3/20

Peter's son David came to our rescue. The shy young boy I had known had grown into a handsome, delightful young man. Qualifying well from an agricultural college in England it had always been his dream to return to the island he loved and have his own farm there, but it was not an easy goal to achieve. He had managed to secure a lease on an old farmhouse, La Ville Farm; the place Ken and I had stayed on our honeymoon.

'You can come and use some of the rooms in the farmhouse if you don't mind roughing it a bit. Perhaps we can come to some agreement?'

So began my new life on Sark. It was still strange to have no real home, but wonderful to be with Peter each day. I missed Roy very much and had to be careful not to try and 'mother' David. I thought he was amazingly mature to accept the odd situation he found himself in: his father living with another woman while his mother accepted the situation. I suspect it was for that very reason David and his sisters accepted me eventually.

We lived like this for a little while, and I wasted no time in discovering if my services as an island nurse would be needed again. The older woman who had been helping was only too pleased to hand over to me, and the then doctor, a delightful Scottish ex-army physician was happy to have me aboard.

My acceptance of people on the Island, after several years away, and the nature of my return, took some time to be accepted. I know there were the inevitable rumours that I had split Peter and Marjorie, but when we three were seen together, that scotched that one.

I had kept up with my 'Sark family' and my godchild Valerie was now a pretty eighteen-year-old, but my old friend Hap had lost an arm in a farming accident. Leaning over an unguarded bailing machine his coat had caught and his arm had been wrenched from its socket and it had to be amputated. If that was not enough, the shock aggravated a latent family predisposition to diabetes and hypertension. He did not take kindly to medication and often refused his treatment.

On my return I was pleased our friendship had not changed, but I was genuine in my concern for the possible effect of his stubbornness. As a trained nurse I knew what the outcome could be.

'I can't be bothered taking all that rubbish, eh.'

'It's not rubbish. It is to stop you having a stroke or worse.'

'Don't care. I'll be out of it then.'

'Huh, well you may not. You may end up with an invalid.' I did not know how prophetic my words would prove to be.

The call came early one morning. 'Auntie Chris,' I could hardly recognise Val's voice; 'it's Pop: he's in hospital in Guernsey; he had a stroke in the night, and he's paralysed all down his right side. Mum's over there now.'

'I'll come round.'

I offered what support I could in the next few days and helped a little in the shop until Annie came back.

'He hasn't had another and the doctor over there says he may be over the worst, but his right side is all paralysed and he can't talk; well except to say 'terna buggre!' Annie looked determined. 'Chris, I want to bring him home. They say he could go on like this for some time, or he might just have another. They won't let me bring him home though, unless I have nursing help...do you think...' I did not wait until she finished.

'He must come home, and I will help as much as I can. We'll need to get some equipment from the St John's in Guernsey.'

Plans were made over the next few days. It was decided to put Hap in the bedroom behind the shop, but there was no bathroom, just a washbasin and toilet.

'We could turn the back storeroom into a bathroom. We'll then be able to keep an eye on him and he'd hear what was going on.' So this is what was done. Sam and Jerry were handy men, and it took no time at all installing a bathroom and widening the doorway.

I had connections with the St John Ambulance and Rescue in Guernsey who had an excellent equipment hire service. I arranged to have a hospital bed, ripple mattress (to prevent bed sores), a commode, mechanical hoist and a bath seat sent to Sark.

Now all we needed was Hap.

When my friend arrived, I was shocked by the change in him. I was expecting the physical change, but the spirit had gone too. I knew this often happened and determined I would get the fight back.

'Well, you old bugger, I warned you this might happen! I've got you at my mercy now.' There was a glint in his eye, and he muttered...'T.t.t.er' and that was the beginning.

He was a mess. With his left arm missing and the right side paralysed, there was only movement in the left leg. A bedsore cut deep into his right heel and there was no control of natural functions. He had a catheter in to relieve his bladder and needed help with everything else. He was a challenge, but I had been used to this sort of case in my nursing days in New Zealand.

Annie was an apt pupil. She had been giving Hap his insulin injections before the stroke, and now he had no choice but to swallow his other medication. I showed her how to roll her father over and sit him up on the edge of the bed, ready to wrap the sling harness round him for the hoist. Hap was not much help and tried to resist till I gave him a good talking to. 'You can be bloody-minded and be difficult and make life hard for everyone, or you can co-operate. Either way we are just as stubborn as you, and we will win.' Hap's power of speech was still limited and consisted of two patois swearwords; 'Terna buggre', which did not need translation, and an explosive 'Te-te-te.' He never said anything else in all the time I helped with his care, as he refused speech therapy. But I have never heard so many ways of saying those few syllables.

At first I visited several times a day. There were many things for the family to learn. They all did their share, but it was on Annie's shoulders the main burden fell. We soon managed to get Hap into the bath on the special seat, using the mechanical hoist. It was a Godsend as we could not have managed the heavy man without. For a while he was in bed all day, and the ripple mattress also was essential to stop bedsores. A small transformer pumped air into alternate cells in the plastic over-mattress, thus relieving the patient's weight on any one spot every few minutes.

The existing bedsore on his right heel was a problem. As a diabetic, the skin healed badly and there was a danger of gangrene. I had been using a wonderfully healing liquid while in New Zealand. It was made from marigolds, called calendula and was known to aid cleansing of wounds and to promote healing. By packing Hap's deep sore twice a day with gauze moistened in this magic liquid, it healed completely.

The other big problem was the catheter. As the stroke had affected natural functions, it was necessary to have a catheter in place permanently. Blockages were frequent and excruciatingly painful for Hap. This often happened in the middle of the night and required swift attention. Sometimes it was possible to unblock it, but more often than not it was necessary to re-catheterise. The first few times the doctor attended, but sometimes he would be out on a call, and poor Hap would be writhing in agony by the time help came.

'I know female nurses are not supposed to catheterise men,' I said to the doctor after one of these occasions, 'which in my mind is ridiculous, but I was trained to do it on my district in New Zealand. Would you let me do it next time?'

'Och, aye,' in his lovely accent, 'I dinna see why not; I'll watch ye the first time, for the record, ye ken.'

I took that on, and became quite expert at the most difficult catheterisation I had ever had to do.

Each day when it was not a bath day, Annie and I would wash Hap. On one of these occasions, a month or so after he returned to Sark, I was lifting his right leg up and it jumped out of my hand.

'Hap, you moved your leg!' I could hardly believe it. I gave him a big hug which brought on an explosion of 'Te-te-te's'. 'You know, we will get you walking if it kills me!'

We did.

It took a lot of effort by all of us. He never managed by himself, but with Annie in the right supporting the bad side and me on the left, he did manage to walk up and down the kitchen. As there was no arm on the left to hook mine into, I had to support him with both my arms wrapped round his torso. He loved that! Many were the saucy looks he gave me and sometimes I had to tell him to concentrate on his walking instead of grinning at me.

With this improvement Hap's attitude changed and he was nearly back to my old antagonist.

3/21

True to my promise the first winter we arranged to bring Roy over from New Zealand, first to visit Sark, see his grandparents, and then we were to meet up with my brother David in a small Swiss village called Saas Fee.

It was wonderful to see my son again. I had wondered if he would hold a grudge, but I did him a disservice. He was his usual loving self. Roy had known Peter when we had run our guest houses and they had always got on well, both having a similar sense of humour.

I had another reason for wanting to get Roy over to the Channel Isles. He was now in the top classes at school in Auckland and wanted to go to university to study computer sciences. The boys' school in Guernsey was particularly good, and I had been to see the headmaster to ask if a place could be found for my son, should he decide to finish his education in the United Kingdom. My brother had gone to Cambridge University and graduated brilliantly. While I did not think Roy was quite in his uncle's league, I knew he was very clever and I wanted the best for him.

'I'm sure you could pass the entrance exam for any of the UK universities. You could visit your father in the summer holidays, and maybe get a seasonal job.'

'It would be winter though, Mum. In any case, there is Annette, my girlfriend: and Dad.' I did not try and persuade Roy: the last thing I wanted to do was divide his loyalties, though I thought, wrongly, his affection for the girlfriend would not last.

'I suppose Ken would be lonely, especially as he said he'd never look at another woman.'

Roy looked a little embarrassed and blushed. 'Er, well, not exactly: you should see some of the women he brings home.' He quickly changed the subject.

We booked a hotel in Saas Fee, near Zermatt. It was a delightful picture-postcard village set in the Swiss Alps. We had all bought 'Moon Boots' and took all our warm clothing, which was needed as the snow was deep throughout the village and surrounding area. The ski lifts started right in the village, and it was not long before David took Roy off for his first lesson.

'You two would be best to try 'Langlauf,' cross-country skiing, it is a bit easier.' Easy or not I found I just could not stay upright. As soon as I got myself in the right position, with poles supporting me, my feet just slid forward, and I landed on my behind each time.

'Huh: too much posterior ballast!' My brother was not much help at all.

Peter managed a little better and stayed upright, but never mastered the art of stopping, except by steering into the nearest snow drift. In the end we settled on long walks in the snow, exploring the local countryside. Roy did very well and seemed to be a 'natural,' much to David's satisfaction.

It was a good holiday, and I was delighted to spend so much time with Roy. It seemed he had not suffered greatly from his parents' separation: he was looking forward to his tertiary education and his own future. I was glad Ken and I had waited until this time instead of when he was younger.

Roy's visit went too quickly, and I was very sad to wave him off at Heathrow Airport, but Peter and I had made plans to visit New Zealand before too long and I had that to look forward to.

In the meantime there was great excitement on Sark. A film company had decided to record a series for television based on a book written by Mervyn Peake. This author and artist had lived on the Island in the 1950s. A group of like-minded friends had accompanied him, and they used a building called the 'Gallery' where they created and displayed their art. The building still stands to this day: now a well-equipped store and Post Office keeping the original name.

To the delight of many of us the cast was world-famous. Mr Pye was played by Derek Jacobi, Miss

Dredger by Judy Parfitt, and Miss George by Betty Marsden. The story told of Mr Pye's visit to Sark to make all the residents Godfearing. By example he was so good he grew wings. To get rid of theses he became badly behaved and started to grow horns. The Island residents tired of his antics and chased him, driving a horse and carriage, all over the Island. He finally flew off the Coupee into the sunrise.

There were many stunts involved, in particular the final chase. This was where I came in. Some time before the arrival of the crew, the Sark doctor had asked if I would be available when dangerous stunts were performed, as there had to be a medical person on site and he was too busy. I had readily agreed, especially as I was being paid, but heard no more so assumed the company had made their own arrangements.

A few days after the filming started, I was helping David remove old plaster from the lounge walls of the old farmhouse: I was covered in dust from head to toe. The phone rang, and then Peter rushed in with a grin on his face.

'That was the filming company: they want you down at the harbour as soon as you can. They are doing a stunt and must have you there.'

I cleaned up as quickly as I could, grabbed my medical bag and hitched a lift on a tractor down the steep harbour hill to see an amazing sight. There was a mock-up of part of 'La Coupe' complete with railings, constructed in the wide area where the tractors normally turned. There also was a black horse and a carriage, with a man standing in it with enormous realistic wings attached to his shoulders. Cameras and crew stood around, and a tractor and trailer with what looked like a pile of mattresses was drawn up close to the far end of the mock-up of 'La Coupee.'

A tall, slim man with a clipboard in his hands hurried over. He quickly introduced himself as the director.

'Good: thanks for coming at such short notice. We thought we had things covered but our medical adviser didn't arrive today.' He looked down at the clipboard. 'You won't have to do anything I hope, but the stunt man has to drive the horse and carriage over the...what do you call it?'

'La Coupee.'

'Yes, La Coupee: through the railings made of polystyrene and jump out of the carriage and onto the pile of mattresses.'

'Yes, right,' I said faintly, 'nothing to it.'

The stunt man set off and had a couple of trial runs.

'Right, now this time jump: O.K?'

The stunt man, who did look a little like Derek Jacobi from a distance, nodded and set off at a gallop. Halfway across he leapt from the moving carriage towards the mattresses...and missed, landing heavily on the edge of the trailer and slipped to the ground. For a second we stood horrified, until I realised I was needed. I rushed over to where the man sat on the ground rubbing his hip.

'Didn't allow for the bloody wings, did I?'

'Don't move for a moment: just want to make sure nothing is broken: you went with an almighty crash.' I felt carefully where he had hit himself and asked him to move his feet and legs. All seemed to be functioning well, but he looked pale and was shaking a little.

'You're in shock. I really think you should rest a little.'

The producer was standing by. 'O.K., Frank, you must go back to the Hotel. I think we got enough shots, anyway.' Turning to me he asked if I could go back with Frank and I agreed.

We got onto the back of the trailer, Frank lying on one of the mattresses and made our way up the Harbour Hill. To my consternation he reached into a side pocket and produced a flask, taking a swig before I could stop him.

'What was that? You know alcohol is not a good idea after an accident!'

'I'll be O.K. It's not the first tumble I've had you know!'

When we got back to the hotel, I helped Frank to his room, and he immediately started to strip off his clothes. It was not until afterwards I realised I could have been in a delicate situation. At the time I concentrated on rubbing Arnica cream thickly on the rapidly darkening bruising on his muscular back and buttocks and getting some ice from the hotel bar for a pack.

'Mmm, that feels good, Nurse…: I don't even know your name?'

'Chris.'

'Well, Chris, I want you around with all my stunts. You know what you are doing!'

It was a fascinating time for everyone involved. The filming crew stayed for a few months and I had several more calls, but none as dramatic as that first one.

The cast and filming crew mixed with the residents: it was impossible not to on such a small Island. I was delighted on one occasion to chat with Derek Jacobi during the filming of a picnic on the beach of Port Du Moulon. We were taking a break and I could not resist the temptation to talk to this actor whom I had admired for years. I had last seen him in a Shakespeare play at the theatre in Stratford-upon-Avon. I was nervous, but felt my uniform gave me some sort of official status.

'This is quite a departure for you, Mr Jacobi: I last saw you in 'The Taming of the Shrew' at Stratford.'

He gave his famous chuckle, and drawled, 'Weell, you know my dear, one has to try new things: don't want to get stagnant.'

'Ha, I can't see that ever happening.' I think I blushed: what a thing to say. I quickly changed the subject and we chatted about Sark. 'It is such a friendly place: and so beautiful. It is like a holiday to be here for this filming.'

I had to agree as I looked up at the towering cliffs, now topped with brilliant yellow gorse in flower. In every crack and ledge wildflowers bloomed. The sea was gently flowing in and out rattling the rounded stones as it moved, and gulls wheeled, crying overhead while the

May sunshine poured down warming everything it touched.

'Yes and I am lucky enough to live here,' I said quietly as I got up to move away as filming started again.

3/22

The rebuilding of Clos des Camps had progressed while I had been preoccupied with the filming, and we decided to move in before it was properly finished. The new building looked very different from the one we had pulled down. Instead of wooden walls, they were solid concrete made to look like granite painted over, with the corner coins of genuine granite showing: it had proved too expensive to have all granite. The walls must have looked realistic as one local man remarked; 'What a shame to paint over that stone-work!'

Soon after the excitement of the filming of famous actors, the island had an even greater visitor. Our new medical centre was to be opened by Queen Elizabeth herself, accompanied by the Duke of Edinburgh.

A Royal visit to Sark was, by most standards, low key. In an Island where crime was practically non-existent and people rarely locked their doors there was little fear of terrorism, but the usual security precautions had to be taken, and day-visitors were restricted. We residents had the unique chance to be very close to the Royal visitors, and I even had a chat with Prince Phillip.

As a nurse I was needed to stand outside the Island Hall in case anyone was taken ill while their Majesties were greeting the local dignitaries inside. Two people were required, so I asked the help of a very attractive young nurse who had come to live on Sark with her family. We were standing to attention in our uniforms by the door when the Queen left the hall, followed a little while afterward by Prince Phillip. Catching sight of my attractive helper, the Prince stopped.

'Oh, I didn't know there were nurses! Are you always here?'

'Well, no sir,' I stammered misunderstanding the comment. 'We don't stay by the hall all the time; we visit homes around the Island.'

'Hm! The Doctor said nothing about you. He must be keeping you to himself, lucky fellow!'

With that the Prince strode to the waiting carriage.

In the meantime, my nursing practice was growing. My care of Hap had overcome most of the adverse gossip...and there was plenty. Novelty of my return had worn off and with residents involved with looking after visitors I could concentrate on settling into my new life. Many of my patients were basic nursing care; help with baths, personal hygiene, even cutting toenails. Home conditions of some residents, particularly the older Sarkese, were not much different from those I had encountered in London, years ago. With no mains water supply or central sewage disposal on the Island, people had to cope as best they could. One elderly couple I visited frequently, mainly to cut toenails and give a vitamin injection, lived in a picturesque place called locally 'Millie's Cottage', after the wife's name, though I later learned it's proper name was 'Le Hurel'...a little rise or hillock.'It was tucked down a no-exit lane and I had no premonition I would be involved there in years to come.

While I enjoyed the basic nursing, I soon became a little frustrated with having little mental stimulation, until one day Peter brought my attention to an advertisement in a national paper.

'Look Chrissie, there is an advert for a correspondence course in Homeopathy...you've been interested in it for ages I know. Why don't you write?'

I did, and so opened a whole new branch to my medical activity.

While much of the work was by correspondence, it was necessary to have consultations with a tutor, and I was lucky to be accepted by a qualified Homeopath in the island of Alderney, the Northern most island in the Channel Isles.

I wrote to the address in the advertisement and in no time I was enrolled as a student for a Diploma with the British Institute of Homeopathy.

It was a very exacting course, involving the purchase of books: essays to be written and marked: visits to Alderney for tutorials, and practical experience. I had become totally unused to the discipline of study, and my tutor told me after I had qualified, she had wondered if I would make it.

'Chris, your first essays were not really up to scratch: but once you got going...well there was no holding you!'

I rediscovered the pleasure of study and had not really thought about having a practice of my own until my tutor suggested I consider it. It had only taken me a year to get my first Diploma, and I was delighted to be made a 'Fellow of the B.I.H' because of my high marks.

'Why not take the advanced Medical Diploma?' My tutor urged, 'I would be happy to be your tutor for that too.' So I took her advice and continued studying for a further two years. It was a much harder course and to be registered at the end, I had to spend a certain time in other homeopathic clinics: sit in on a set number of consultations and write 25 case studies.

I had thought Peter would be unhappy about my being away for two weeks, as he hated me to be away without him. We had become even closer over the years, and I loved being with him, but he was inclined to be a little possessive. When I tackled him once, his reply floored me; 'Well, Chris, you left Ken, you might do the same to me, and I couldn't bear that.'

I put my arms tightly round him and promised that would never happen, but I knew deep down he was still insecure. There was much of the 'little boy' about Peter: as I loved him so much it did not matter to me if he always wanted me by his side.

That was why I was surprised when he helped me arrange a visit to relatives of his in England.

'I have approached my cousin Evelyn and her husband Don, in Dover. I think you said there are several clinics near there you can attend, so you could stay with them. I can pop over at the weekends maybe?'

Staying with Peter's relatives, I had two weeks of travelling to various homeopathic clinics in the area. As I had kept my little Fiat car in England with Peter's daughter Lynn, I had transport. Clinics were held at all hours, and by driving from one to another, with sometimes a twelve-hour day, I managed to accumulate the necessary hours of experience.

It was November, and the weather was as grey and drizzly as only an English November can be, but I enjoyed the clinics and meeting other homeopaths. One has remained my friend for many years.

Soon after my return to Sark I realised I wanted to put my knowledge into practice. My exposure to the clinics in the U.K. reinforced my belief in total care of a patient. Throughout my nursing experience I had time and again acknowledged the need to look beyond the medical diagnosis. In taking a homeopathic consultation the practitioner studies every aspect of the patient, from past family history, dietary preferences, sleep and dream patterns, emotional states, and bodily functions. During the one and a half hour first consultation, a homeopath will be observing behaviour and appearance and reaction to questioning. At the end, a full picture will emerge; a medical diagnosis is not necessarily of prime importance. Treatment centres around strengthening the person's immune system, so the body can fight the medical or emotional problem.

It was my experience over the many years I practiced, much of the help came from the intimate long consultation, where often patients would remark, 'I never told anyone that before.' It was my aim to have a relaxed, comfortable person before I even thought of a remedy which would help the physical or mental problems. Half the healing would already have begun. My experiences as a district nurse in New Zealand, and a course on counselling were of great value.

After I had taken other courses including two years of herbal medicine, I formed my 'Healthy Life Clinics' in

Sark and Guernsey. These covered lifestyle advice, diet control, homeopathy, and hair root analysis from a specialist doctor in Wimpole St in London.

As soon as I was fully qualified, I realised I would need somewhere to practice. Sark was not a problem, but it took me some time to find the ideal place in Guernsey. At first I was offered partial use of a shop at the top of one of the steep winding cobbled streets in the main town of St Peter Port. As I walked up the old, cobbled streets, I remembered reading Elizabeth Gouge's '*Green Dolphin Country*' set in Guernsey and New Zealand. She wrote of the swirling, buffeting wind skittering down the lanes, and I was transported back a century. The wooden shopfronts could hardly have changed since that day, and as I approached the one which would be my first clinic rooms, my heart skipped a beat. There was a large, bowed window facing down the hill, with green-painted woodwork. It did not look like a clinic, but when I put up some copies of my certificates and a notice, it looked more authentic.

I had taken my first steps into a new profession.

3/23

It was hard work at first and the shop was not ideal. I had to buy a screen to give some privacy from the passers-by, and there was no waiting area. If my next patients arrived before I had finished the previous one, they had to stand outside. It was a very quiet part of town and as I sometimes gave an evening consultation, I felt a little vulnerable.

This was brought home on one occasion when I had made an appointment one evening for a young man who said he worked during the day. When this happened, I usually stayed in a small bed and breakfast place nearby as there were no evening boats back to Sark.

When the patient arrived, I became a little alarmed. He was shaven headed, with tattoos and piercings, but his manner was quite pleasant.

As usual I started my consultation by asking my patient what he felt was his problem.

'Well, I have just come out of prison...a little drug misunderstanding, you might say.' I sat uncomfortably twiddling my pen thinking I could be in trouble and wondered how quickly I could reach the door.

'I want to do better with my life: my sister Jenny you saw a couple of months ago, said you did wonders for her. She nagged me to come and see you.' He sat with his arms folded.

'Well, what do you think I can do? Do you want to get off drugs?'

'I'm just about clean now, but I get these night sweats and a rash.'

Now we were talking my language and gradually I took a history, realising he was the same as all my other patients. He needed reassurance and support as much as medication. As with all my patients I told him he could phone me if he needed to talk; he did on a regular basis for nearly six months. Gradually this young man improved, then went to night school to study social work.

The last I heard he was working among drug addicts in the East End of London.

It may not have been pure homeopathy, but it worked.

Over the thirteen years I ran my 'Healthy Life Clinic' I moved to a combined clinic out of the main centre, and then I had a stroke of luck with one of my younger patients. She was pregnant and had come to me for a little advice about vitamin supplements.

'You know, Chris, you'd be better in St Peter Port, and I know just the place.' She went on to tell me she had been attending the Family Planning Rooms right in the main street, "The Pollet."

'They are looking for other people to rent rooms, if you are interested.'

I arranged to book a regular day and my practice increased. With a waiting room, toilet, and small kitchen, it was ideal. Whole families came to see me, and I had several major successes; particularly working with patients' doctors. Pure Homeopaths decry vaccinations, but I had enough medical knowledge to work out a compromise. It was possible to treat young children with homeopathy so that when they had their vaccinations, side effects were mostly avoided. I think part of my success was due to my medical background; patients knew I had experience and could see both sides of a problem.

I was particularly delighted to have children as patients. I felt I had a chance to set them up for a healthy life. One family I became very attached to. There were three little boys; John aged eight, Terry aged five and little two-year-old Jack. The two older brothers had diagnosed Asperger's syndrome, but Jack was too young yet to determine if he was also going to be affected. Their mother, Tina, had founded a help group and together we worked on a treatment for the two delightfully bright boys. One interesting discovery was how they improved when their diets were changed. One very toxic ingredient was orange colouring in some of the drinks and foods.

She variously tried reducing dairy and wheat products and keeping to small frequent, healthy meals devoid of additives. Gradually the behaviour of John and Terry improved and to my delight one day they both climbed on my knee.

This was an achievement, as one of the particulars of Asperger's was a dislike of personal contact and being touched.

I made a big mistake with another older girl with the same diagnosis. We had progressed quite well, and she had made some improvement, until one day as she was leaving the consulting room I touched her on the shoulder in encouragement. She shrunk away from my hand and bolted through the door while I chided myself at my mistake.

On other occasions my medical knowledge was helpful but not always accepted. One day a man came in with his young son who had an ear infection. I suggested he really should see a doctor, but he said, 'I have heard Homeopathy is effective, so we'll see...' I prescribed a couple of remedies but was not too happy about this. A few days later I telephoned, and he was quite irate saying it hadn't worked and he had to go to his doctor in the end. 'Just proved Homeopathy is no good.' I had to bite my tongue not to make the obvious retort.

In other cases my medical knowledge was tested by the effectiveness of certain Homeopathic and Complementary treatments.

I often took the chance of attending a seminar or course of lectures in UK, and one which particularly interested me was based on a 'Sequential therapy.' In this, the practitioner takes a 'timeline' of all illnesses and treatments of the patient. There was a certain formula, starting from the most recent ailment of 'detoxing' item by item, using certain specific Homeopathic remedies. If successful, each illness or medication was pulled to the fore and the toxicity which was always left behind was removed. In this process often a crisis was created, and to heal this there was a formula of four remedies... I called it my Homeopathic Prozac...which was very effective.

This was quite a lengthy and sometimes traumatic process, and not for the faint-hearted, so I chose my patients with care.

One such was a woman of seventy who had a history of thrombosis, pneumonia and legionnaire's disease, and many courses of antibiotics. When I met her she had little energy and seldom left the house. By the time we had worked through half of her timeline, she was driving her car again and visiting friends she had not seen for some time. Her hug and thanks were well worth the hours of treatment and telephone calls.

The discovery of my 'Homeopathic Prozac' proved to have a side use when I had requests sometimes from patients to wean themselves off anti-depressants.

Working with their doctors it was very successful.

My clinics in Guernsey were mostly set for a Wednesday when there was the 'shopping trip.' As I booked ahead, of course I had to make every effort to travel over the often wildly churning sea. As I was such a bad sailor, I blessed Bach Rescue Remedy time and time again in helping me to retain my breakfast. I remembered how it had calmed my friend Allie's fractious sheep all those years previously.

Seeing patients in Sark was easy in comparison. Very often I would leave treatment at May's shop and collect the payment later. Consultations were often in people's homes. Many of the Sarkese had inherited their ancestors' interest in herbal medicine so my practice was not so far from their knowledge, and I learned a few tips on the way.

3/24

When I returned to Sark and became the Island Nurse again, a Scottish retired Air force doctor was holding the position. He was a lovely man, but I often had to ask twice for his telephone instructions as his accent was difficult for me to understand, though I had lived in Edinburgh as a child. He was not much practiced on 'women's' problems, so I had plans to hold special clinics for women. He retired before I could organise anything and the new doctor, Mitch, was an obstetrician as well as experienced in minor surgery.

Soon after his arrival he asked me to call in to his home. We had already met, and I liked him very much.

'Chris, I am in a bit of a spot. I need to go to the dentist next week and wondered if you could stand in for me?' I had been in touch with the Royal College of Nursing who were responsible for my insurance cover, regarding responsibilities outside a nurse's normal experience.

The reply stated: *'As long as you do not diagnose or prescribe, and you have contact with a qualified doctor, we do not see a problem.'* So, I was able to say I was happy to help.

This was to be a 'baptism of fire.'

Although it was not the busiest holiday season there were several day visitors on the Island. As there are no cars on Sark, many people delighted in hiring bicycles and exploring the lanes and footpaths. Some of these paths were not suitable for cycling, particularly when ridden by inexperienced people. My first casualty was one such ill-advised lady who did just that, falling heavily on her shoulder and knee on a steep footpath.

The system for dealing with casualties was well organised. If a patient needed to go to the hospital in Guernsey the St John's very fast ambulance launch, 'The Flying Christine' was sent. The medical person in charge in Sark phoned the St John headquarters: explained the circumstances and was told the expected time the ambulance launch would arrive at Maseline Harbour. The Sark volunteer ambulance men were then alerted to collect the patient in the tractor-drawn ambulance and to arrive at the harbour to meet the launch.

In this, and in subsequent occasions, the St John Headquarters had been alerted by our doctor I was acting as locum. A doctors' surgery in Guernsey had also been informed I was on call, and I could contact them for advice if necessary: this was the days before mobile phones. In later years it was much easier, and I could contact our doctor directly.

As soon as I was alerted about this accident, I rushed to the site taking my, and the doctor's, medical bag. I also collected a blanket as I suspected some major problem as the patient was said to be screaming with pain and unable to move.

I had taken several advanced first aid certificates, and it did not take long to realise the lady had broken her collar bone and dislocated her knee. I gave what first aid I could and sent someone to phone our ambulance. When they arrived, I ran home as it was not far away, and phoned the St John. Within an hour of my seeing her, the unfortunate lady was in the Guernsey Hospital.

I was amused when I reported to Mitch on his return, to hear his story. The dentist's surgery had a wonderful view from above the harbour and over to Sark and Herm. He happened to glance out of the window from the dentist's chair and was horrified to see the ambulance launch making for Sark.

'Chris I was wondering what on earth had happened. At least my concern and distraction made the dentist's efforts less unpleasant.'

Over the years this excellent doctor practiced on Sark, I was to be summoned on many occasions to stand in for him, sometimes overnight. He usually left a note on the surgery door saying he would be back the next day, but in an emergency to phone me.

On one of those occasions the Island constable phoned me in some agitation. 'Old Fred was out with one of the drivers and has collapsed: Chris can you come and see him?'

'Where is he?'

'We drove to the surgery; realised you were on call and unharnessed the horse: he's still on the carriage.'

I knew the old Sarkee well, as he was one of the Island's characters. Too old and frail to drive by himself now, his wife used to let him go out with a younger driver, theoretically 'instructing' the young woman although she was fully qualified. Thus they preserved his dignity and could keep an eye on him.

I did not like the look of the old man as soon as I clambered onto the carriage. The absence of a pulse confirmed my suspicion. 'I think he's dead,' I whispered to the constable, not wanting to alarm the inevitable bystanders.

'So do I', the constable whispered back.

'I think we had better harness up the horse and take him home. Can someone quickly go and warn his wife, please?'

As we approached the old farmhouse, the man's wife rushed out. 'Are you sure he's dead. Sorry, but you are only a nurse. I must have a doctor! Someone go and get the retired doctor. You must try to revive him!'

Protest as I might she insisted the patient was carried into their bedroom and nothing would satisfy her but that I give mouth to mouth resuscitation. I shall never forget the sensation of the cold lips on mine and the breath I blew in nauseatingly seeping out as I bent to give another breath.

The retired doctor, who apparently was a friend, arrived soon and confirmed my diagnosis.

Other incidents caused some amusement. There was the time the wife of a local dignitary phoned and asked for help in having a bath.

'Chris, I've cracked my ribs and am having difficulty, could you pop round, do you think?'

I agreed and asked what had happened.

'Don't laugh: I fell in a grave!' I tried not to laugh and went to help the unfortunate lady.

I got the story as we sat having a cup of tea after I had helped with the bath.

'Well, I was standing at the dug grave to drop in a flower.' She took a sip of tea and winced as she moved to set the cup down; 'you know our old gardener died? Thought he'd like that: I turned round to follow everyone who'd already gone into the church and slipped on the wet grass.' She picked up her cup and took another swallow and gave a grimace; 'Before I knew what had happened, I found myself at the bottom of the grave on my back.'

'How on earth did you get out? They could have lowered the coffin on top of you.'

'Exactly my thoughts: I yelled blue murder and fortunately I had been missed and they came and hauled me out. Felt such a fool!'

Her husband had just come into the room. With a grin he sat down opposite his wife.

'Bet it's the first time any of your patients came out of the grave, Chris.'

3/25

As time went by, I had more and more nursing to do which was very satisfying. Added to this, when Mitch knew I had worked in a minor ops theatre years ago in London, he asked me to assist him on occasion. He only performed operations under local anaesthetic, but it saved residents the expense and inconvenience of having to travel to Guernsey. I delighted once more in 'theatre routine' involving setting up and assisting the procedure and sterilising the instruments afterwards; we worked well together.

Peter was happy for me to be nursing again but there were times when I was on call for the doctor, he sometimes was not too keen for me to accept: especally if it conflicted with any plans we had made. I know it was partly because I became anxious when I was 'on call' as it was such a responsibility and I 'switched to my nursing mode', as he put it, being more abrupt and a little distracted. I had reason to be anxious, as a nursing friend in Guernsey pointed out; despite my Royal College of Nursing insurance cover I was very vulnerable to litigation.

This was brought home to me in no uncertain way during one overnight 'on call' session. A middle-aged lady, living with her sister in Little Sark had a fall at home and I was asked to see her. I knew the woman was prone to confusion, but her reactions and state concerned me when I examined her.

By this time the doctor had a mobile phone, so I contacted him and said I thought she should go on the ambulance launch to the Guernsey hospital.

'Oh, Chris; she is always falling, and you know she has mild dementia. Leave it to the morning and see how she is.'

I was not happy but went by the doctor's decision, but early next morning the sister phoned in distress.

'Chris I am so worried; Fanny fell again and I can't rouse her.' I was there as fast as my bike would take me: even riding part-way across La Coupee which was discouraged.

There was no doubt the patient was much worse, so I ordered an ambulance and told the doctor afterwards.

The patient died in the hospital from a subdural haemorrhage.

Soon afterwards the doctor asked me to call into the surgery and I was alarmed to see a policeman from Guernsey with him.

'It's alright, Chris: don't worry, but you will need to make a statement for the coroner. There was a lot of scarring on her brain from previous falls, so it was just a matter of time before this happened.'

I wrote the whole story down as it had occurred, and there were no repercussions: but it caused me a few sleepless nights and I had to think seriously about my situation. I think the doctor was concerned for me too, as I was not asked so often to take an overnight 'locum' after that.

I had several other patients I thoroughly enjoyed seeing. One very elderly lady became a 'regular.' She was not keen on calling a doctor, so whenever she had a problem, I would get a phone call.

'Hello, Christine: when you are next down this way could you just call in, do you think, please?' She was from a wealthy family and was reserved about her personal female problems. She had a recurring discomfort which I was able to relieve. After treatment we developed a ritual.

'Do join me for a sherry my dear:' which would be brought to us on a silver tray in crystal glasses, in the garden in summer, and in the beautifully furnished lounge during the winter in front of a roaring log fire.

They were a couple from the old school and still called each other by their unabbreviated Christian names. After many years of devoted marriage, the husband developed dementia or Alzheimer's disease as we now call it. I would get calls at all hours of day and night to help persuade the old man, dressed only in his pyjamas, to come in from the garden. He loved to wander through the lawns and glades, and when he finally died his widow laid him to rest in one of his favourite places in the garden.

'Well, Christine, there is no law to say I cannot do that, is there?'

I felt it was a privilege to serve these Island residents and sometimes they were people I had known since my guest house days in the 1960s. I was on the boat back to Sark one day after a homeopathic surgery, and her niece, a friend who now lived in Guernsey, came over to sit with me.

'Chris, I've been meaning to ask you. You may know Auntie Heather has cancer...'

'Yes I had heard: I am so sorry: she was always such a livewire.'

'Yes, well: she won't come over to Guernsey for me to look after her. She is determined to stay at home.'

I thought of the old cottage Heather lived in with outside sanitation and water collected from a tap in the yard. I knew her daughter lived in Jersey and was soon expecting her first child.

I was concerned with what I guessed was coming but had to ask. 'What do you want me to do?'

'Could you keep an eye on her, d'you think? She can look after herself now and people go in to take food and so on, but I can't stay over there: I have my boys to think of.'

I already had several patients on daily visits, but I could only say 'yes.' Heather and her husband had been our 'carters' when my husband Ken and I arrived new to the Island. They had helped us settle in, delivering groceries and collecting guests' luggage. After her husband's death Heather had valiantly carried on the carting and carriage business.

For several weeks I called in when I could to check Heather was coping, and at first she managed to feed her geese and look after herself. I hated the geese chasing me across her front yard and used to amuse Heather when I dived into the cottage, slamming the door against their ferocious beaks.

'They'll get you one day, Chris.'

As I became less busy with other patients and to get Heather used to me in a more intimate way, I tried to stay a little longer in my visits. I knew the time was approaching when my patient would need more personal care.

One day as we were sitting by the fire sipping our cups of coffee, Heather suddenly laughed. 'You know, Chris you caused quite a stir when news came that you and Peter Curtis were going to live together. The stories I heard...!'

'What do you mean?'

'Oh, that Curtis had met a nurse in New Zealand, and she has seduced him and pushed his wife Marjorie out of their marriage.'

I felt a little sick. I had no idea of those stories and was thankful I had not known when I returned to Sark: I doubt otherwise whether I would have had the courage.

'Well, of course, when I heard your name, I had to chuckle: and anyway everyone knew that the Curtis' were not getting along too well. After all, he was living in the little cottage and she was in the main house.'

Not for the first time I was aware of the power of gossip on this small island. I had noticed one or two cold receptions from people I had known before but thought little of it at the time.

'Anyway, you stuck it out and a good thing for Sark is all I can say.'

I reached over and squeezed Heather's hand. I was fond of this gutsy lady and was very sad she would not be with us much longer: I was determined to keep her at home as she wanted, if at all possible.

Heather's deterioration was rapid, and soon she was unable to leave her bed for long. I managed to visit twice a day, often needing to light the fire and get her some breakfast before boiling water and giving her a wash. But she was content, and people called in to keep her company. Her niece from Guernsey came over as often as she could and when I was expecting her I tended to miss the afternoon visit.

One day I shall not forget.

I visited in the morning as usual, but as her niece was going to spend the afternoon with Heather and I had several other patients, I said I would not call.

'Please Chris, do pop in if you can: there is something...' She had to stop with a coughing fit. I patted her hand and said I would try.

I did not manage to visit, and it was the last time I saw Heather alive. She died that night.

When I called to perform last offices...something I regularly did...Heather's niece was still there. She handed me a package: 'Auntie wanted to give this to you herself, but just didn't make it. I brought it over yesterday.'

Inside the package was an engraved picture of geese, running with beaks outstretched and wings wide. Underneath she had had inscribed 'Watch out for your heels Chrys.'

It has remained one of my prized possessions, complete with the miss-spelling of my name.

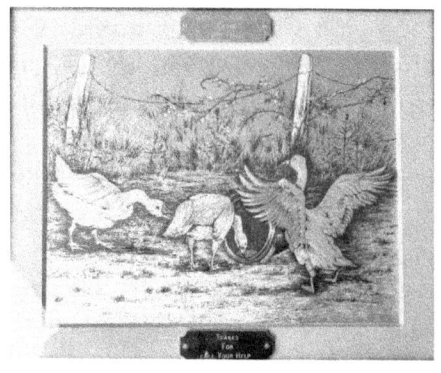

3/26

Apart from people referred by the doctor, I could take on patients by my own choice but usually I checked with him first. Occasionally I had to act as an intermediary as they would not consult the doctor. I would receive a phone call...often in the night...which went something like; 'I don't want to bother the doctor, but I wonder if you would just come and see my mother/husband/ child.'

The call I had from Mavis was just such a one. We had occasionally invited Mavis and her sister Hagar for a meal and found their stories from the Second World War intriguing. The family had been in Singapore when it fell and had just escaped in time. The ship they were on was bombed and the two young children and their parents were interned but they were all united and had moved to Sark many years ago. I do not know whether it was their experiences, or they had embraced it before, but they belonged to a religious sect with certain peculiarities; one of which was a distrust of doctors and hospitals.

Hence their phone call to me.

'Chris; we are a little worried about Mother. She had a fall and is complaining her hip really hurts when she moves.'

My first thought was a possible fractured neck of femur, all too common in the elderly after a fall, and was concerned about their need of a doctor's visit let alone hospitalisation and an operation.

As I pulled on my waterproof jacket and leggings I was not looking forward to a cycle ride to Little Sark and a trip over La Coupe, for it had just started to hail and the wind was making up to gale force. Trying not to think of the evening I had planned with Peter in front of our log fire after a pleasant meal, I strapped my bag on the carrier and mounted my trusty bike. I was quite sheltered by the banks by the road until I approached the high isthmus of the Coupe. Then the elements attacked me as I walked across and tried to mount again. I just could not get on the bike or even make progress walking, as the rough wind and hail kept pushing me nearer and nearer the edge. In exasperation I shouted, 'Stop pushing me about will you,' and my anger gave me enough energy to make it to the gateway of my patient's house.

Here I discovered, as I had suspected, the old lady had a possible fracture. I knew the pain in the hip radiating into the groin was a known symptom, as was the slight out turning of her foot.

'I'm sorry, but you must have the doctor attend, Mavis. I think Mother has broken her hip.'

'Will it heal?'

'Sorry, not by itself; she will need an operation.'

'Oh, I don't know. We don't believe in any of that.' Turning to her sister, she said, 'Let's talk to Father.'

I was totally bemused as I knew their father had died several years ago and could not resist the temptation of peeping through the open door as the two sisters went into the next room. There on the mantelpiece was an ornate urn, the sort used for storing mortal ashes and the women were addressing it.

I quickly went back to the old lady, trying to make her more comfortable, until they returned.

'We would rather you came back in the morning. We don't think Father would like it...''

I could hear a gust of wind and the rattle of hail against the window and my patience was wearing thin. I was not prepared to take the responsibility of a worsening condition. Then I had an idea as I knew they had a religious leader in Guernsey, and so insisted they phone him.

I explained the situation and he was sympathetic, agreeing under those circumstances the old lady should have any medical help she needed so I asked him to inform Mavis.

The doctor arrived and confirmed my suspicions, but the weather was too rough to get the ambulance launch over until the morning when the forecast was for a drop in the wind. I made the old lady as comfortable as I could by packing her firmly with pillows and gratefully swung my bicycle on the doctor's tractor to have a ride home.

A glass of ginger wine and a sympathetic hug from Peter restored my sanity; until the phone rang at seven the next morning.

'Chris, I think Mother is better and no need to go over to Guernsey.'

Groaning, I peddled back to their house, grateful the wind had indeed moderated, and a weak sun was trying to make amends for the hail of the previous evening.

The old lady had slept well and looked better, but I was not convinced as she tried to pull herself up the bed and said,

'I want to pass water.'

There was a commode by the bed, and I tried to be as gentle as possible, but the poor soul screamed as I lifted her out. I had little satisfaction in being right and stayed until the Sark ambulance arrived at nine thirty, wondering if I would see her again. Post operative shock was a killer in such cases, and the old lady was very frail.

I was wrong.

After a few weeks, Mother came back but was not able to walk. I reluctantly agreed to help with the nursing, thinking her two able bodied daughters were more than capable. I hoped eventually they would see to her hygiene and comfort with just a little advice from me, as I had several ill patients. For some time they could be seen pushing Mother, wrapped up like a mummy, in a wheelchair and the rumour circulated she had died already and they were wheeling a cadaver about. Having witnessed the consultation of Father's ashes I could have been excused for believing this if I had not been attending occasionally. Gradually the old lady became weaker, and I really felt she needed full-time care, especially as I started to receive calls, often at night, to lift Mother onto the commode as Mavis said she could not mange on her own.

'What about Hagar?'

'I didn't want to wake her. She needs her sleep.' As a diagnosed schizophrenic I had to accept that, but the final straw came when I arrived in the middle of the night to be told.

'She says she doesn't want to go to the toilet now.'

I had never refused a patient before, but I could see my life being governed more and more by these strange women, and insisted they employ a full-time carer.

Amazingly the old woman hung on for another year, and I supposed she had eventually gone to join her husband on Mavis and Hagar's mantelpiece, to be consulted by their dutiful daughters at every crisis.

As such, the parents had gained a certain immortality.

3/27

With the passing years, the doctor and his lovely wife had become friends with Peter and me. Gradually Anthea had changed the fenced-in corner of a field where the new Medical Centre and their house stood, to a beautiful garden and as I was a keen gardener we had a lot in common.

Anthea and I sometimes chatted on the phone, so I was not altogether surprised when she rang me at seven one morning as I knew they were usually early risers.

'Oh, Chris, can you come round. Mitch thinks he's had a heart attack.'

I quickly dressed and raced round to the Medical Centre which was not far away.

Mitch certainly looked very ill and I did not need to see his ECG which he had taken, to realise there had been a cardiac incident. Together we arranged the St John ambulance launch to collect him, and for his entry to the hospital in Guernsey.

'You'll need to contact the Seigneur and the Medical Committee: they will have to arrange a locum: do you think you can hold the fort?'

'That's OK: don't you worry, we'll arrange something. Just get well.'

It was a while before Mitch was allowed to return: heart surgery and aftercare were necessary. In the meantime, the Sark Medical Committee contacted several doctors in Guernsey who had acted as locum in the past when Mitch and Anthea went away on holiday.

I was asked to look after the practice in between doctors. As it was peak holiday time, I was kept pretty busy, but fortunately there were no major incidents like carriage accidents: a not unknown occurrence. One locum was a retired cardiac specialist and used to say visits to Sark were a 'rest-cure.' He normally came in the winter when Mitch and Anthea preferred to go away for some winter sun. On this occasion the specialist came over to

Sark on the August Bank Holiday: one of the busiest weekends in the year.

He called me in to do a few visits, and I was amused by his comment:

'I'll never rib Mitch again: I've never been so rushed. I didn't realise how much was involved here: not only two surgeries each day, but all your own dispensing and being on call 24 hours a day! We Guernsey doctors thought this was a cushy number.'

Eventually our lovely doctor returned to us, but he had to be careful and have an annual check-up in England. I was always a little concerned for him if we had an emergency call out together as sometime occurred. Once we were called to attend the collapse of a visitor in one of the shops. We both arrived at the same time, and we could see she was in a bad way. Customers had been cleared and the shop closed as Mitch knelt by the woman's side and tried for a pulse.

'Can't find one Chris; CPR: you do the respiration and I'll do the heart.'

For what seemed like forever we laboured, and at last I found a faint flutter in the carotid artery, but had one eye on Mitch, praying he would not collapse as well. After the patient had gone to Guernsey on the Ambulance launch he looked at me with an eyebrow raised. 'I could see you had one eye on me Chris!'

It was Anthea who was to be a casualty before her husband.

On one of Mitch's annual check-ups, she mentioned she had not been feeling very well and the heart specialist gave her a thorough examination. What they found had her straight into hospital for an operation as she had advanced arteriosclerosis. My happy bright friend never really recovered fully and had a massive stroke during a cruise with Mitch a few years later.

The shock made me very aware of how fragile life could be, and I valued even more the life I had on this lovely Island. The thought of a future without Peter, the man I had learned to love so much, made me almost sick with panic. There was a lot of laughter in my life as he told so many jokes and was so full of energy and exuberance. I tried not to think about something I knew I could not control, although it was constantly in my prayers. While I would not call myself 'religious,' I have felt a presence throughout my life and firmly believe in a loving, though not predictable God. At a risk of seeming casual, I have been prone to 'arrow prayers:' a sort of one-sided conversation on my part.

I sometimes found myself in the Island's Church, St Peter's when there was no-one else there and the arrow prayers were constantly launched from my heart. Besides attending choir practice each Thursday and Church on Sundays, every few weeks Peter and I had undertaken to be on the 'Church-opening' roster. This responsibility came about as a result of the current Vicar living some distance from the church. So it was that we volunteered to collect the large cast-iron key in the morning to open the church and lock it up at night. It was not an onerous duty, and as there were at least six people on the roster, we were not called upon often. In summer we opened quite early and closed later at night. I used to love the silence of the early and late hours, disturbed only by a distant bird's call or the clip-clop of a horse going by. I felt a deep peace settle into my heart, and my arrow prayers would be ones of thanks.

There were a few amusing times: suddenly getting ready for bed and one of us asking: 'Did you lock the church?' Followed by a very un-Christian exclamation; a quick pulling on of jeans over night attire and a moonlit cycle-ride quickly to do the job.

Once I arrived to lock up, and just checked to make sure no-one was inside. There was a lady sitting in a pew, bowed over apparently in prayer: I cycled round the block: she was still at prayer. After the third circuit I ventured into the church and cleared my throat: she started up, blushing.

'Oh, dear, I must have dropped off: it is so peaceful here!'

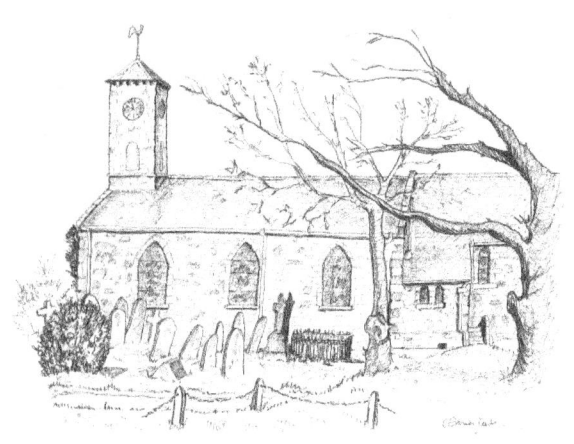

St Peters Church, Sark

3/28

One of the delights of my new life in Sark was the frequent holidays Peter and I were able to take. My dear mother had died and left a substantial legacy, and Peter was in a 'comfortable' financial position, as he put it, when we were settled in the rebuilt Clos des Camps.

'Chrissie, we will have lots of trips. We both were unable to travel when we had our guest houses, so we will make up for it now.' Wrapping me in his bear hug of an embrace, he continued; 'Can't think of a better way to spend my money with you!'

We visited New Zealand every three years to catch up with Roy and Peter's relatives. In between we had Safaris in Kenya, Zimbabwe and Tanzania; trips to the Seychelles, Tobago, Canada and America and a wonderful 'Round the World Trip'. For the first several years Peter had been his usual bouncy self, but once in Canada he had complained of a tingling in his left arm and sinus trouble, but we had thought nothing of it.

Each time we had long air flights, Peter seemed less resilient, and in the year 2000 during our visit to New Zealand he was not his self at all.

'The blessed air conditioning on the plane just doesn't suit me.' But I was a little worried: I had to remind myself that he was now 70 years old, and the brightness had dimmed.

'You are going to have a good check-up when we get home: no putting it off this time.'

As before, Peter seemed a little better when we were back on Sark, and he did not go to see the doctor straight away. He could be pretty stubborn at times.

'I'll go when Mitch comes back from his cruise; don't like that new locum.'

Quite suddenly things got worse. For anyone else I would have noticed earlier, but when you are close to someone you love, it is hard to see the signs. He started to veer to one side when we went for a walk and tired easily, but it was not until Peter kept dropping his fork while eating, I realised there was something very wrong.

I took him to see the locum: but not knowing Peter, he said he would wait and see, and send him in a few days to Guernsey if he was no better. In a couple of days he was worse, and so I phoned the doctor to call as Peter was unable to walk to the surgery.

'Mmm: I think you must go over today and have a scan. I'll order the ambulance.' The doctor said little, but I suspected TIAs (Transitional Ischaemic Attacks), which would account for the symptoms.

I was not prepared for the comments of the specialist in Guernsey, after the scan.

'I am sorry Mrs Curtis: there is a shadow in the left frontal lobe. I don't like the look of it: you will have to go to Southampton as soon as possible.' I still did not realise the significance of what was being said. I suppose my mind would not accept the possibility of a growth.

We booked into a hotel in Guernsey and spent an unreal evening of luxury. Peter seemed completely calm and unconcerned: child-like almost. I was just stunned at the speed of the change in our lives.

I had packed a small case for both of us, expecting just one night away, but in the event, it was several days of nightmare before we returned to Sark.

I remember little of the flight to Southampton and the taxi ride to the hospital. Peter was expected and admitted to a small side-room in a busy general ward. He showed a little of his old spark when he insisted he had health insurance and expected private treatment. I had at last realised the seriousness and phoned his daughter Lynn, who was very close to her father.

'Chris, I'll come right away.' She arrived on the day they decided to operate on Peter and do a biopsy.

I am not sure if the surgeon was annoyed at Peter's attitude, was over-worked, or just insensitive, but I will never forgive him for the way he gave us the devastating news after the operation.

In the centre of the busy ward he just announced to Lynn and me:

'The biopsy showed that Mr Curtis has an advanced astrocytoma. It is inoperable; we removed some fluid which will give temporary relief, but it is terminal. A few months: maybe a year.'

I felt as if my brain would burst; the world stood still for a moment, and I had to support myself on the wall as dizziness overtook me. Lynn looked as stunned as I felt.

A passing nurse must have seen our distress and held my elbow. 'Are you alright, Mrs Curtis?' Anger took over.

'No of course I am not alright. I've just been told the man I love may die in a few months. Your surgeon is the most insensitive doctor I have ever met...and I've worked with a few.'

Lynn was recovering a little; as a social worker she was a sensible and practical woman.

'We want to talk to the surgeon again: now.'

As we went towards Peter's ward we agreed to say nothing to him. 'Maybe there is something that can be done?'

The nurse must have spoken to the doctor and said how distressed we were, as he arrived in Peter's ward soon after we did. Peter was still sleepy from the operation and was oblivious of all round him.

The surgeon took us into the nurses' office this time; he was a little contrite at his earlier insensitivity. 'I thought you would have realised what the diagnosis was likely to be as you are a nurse. I am sorry if it was a shock. I assumed they had told you in Guernsey.'

'No: but surely something can be done?'

'An operation to remove it is impossible as it is well attached to the brain but maybe radiotherapy may delay things a bit. I'll get in touch with Dr Wells, head of radiotherapy.'

With that we had to be content. We were still suffering from shock. I realised I should have suspected some brain problem: the constant ache to Peter's face: his tingling hand: some unusual behaviour over the past year or so, such as repeating certain words and being unconcerned about problems in his work which would normally have annoyed him. As I had said to Lynn, it is difficult to see when you are so close to someone you love.

Dispassionately, I realised I was going through the stages of grief as described by Doctor Kubler-Ross I had observed so many times in families of terminal patients: denial: anger: bargaining: depression and acceptance. I was determined not to accept there was nothing that could be done. Dr Wells arrived later that day and took us to a quiet place. He was the opposite in behaviour to his colleague.

'First let me say how sorry that you have had this news; but as far as...Peter, is it....is concerned, he will not suffer. I will say that if I was told I was going to have cancer, it is the one that I would choose. No pain, just gradually slipping away, and not really knowing what was happening.'

'Surely there is something to be done?'

'Well, yes, I think we could try making a mould to isolate the area in the right temporal region where the tumour is and zapping it with radio waves. I'll prescribe some steroids to try and reduce the collection of fluid. You are a nurse, I believe Mrs Curtis?'

I nodded, unable to trust my voice.

'We will put him on a highish dose and then reduce it in stages. You will know what to look for while he is on the treatment.'

I had to ask the inevitable question.

'How long have we got?'

'It is never sure: maybe six months: if you are lucky and he responds, maybe two years, but it is pretty advanced.'

'Does that mean he has had it there for a long time?'

'Probably for years: but it would have made no difference to the outcome had it been diagnosed earlier, as it is inoperable. Sometimes these growths just sit there till the person dies naturally: sometimes something triggers it to start growing.'

I thought back to our time together, totally unsuspecting this thing had been sitting there in Peter's brain like an alien implant. I wondered how we would have felt had we known it was there: waiting to discover if it would grow or not.

We discussed the treatment, and in the practicalities, I buried my grief.

'It will be a three-month treatment: about a half to one hour each weekday. Peter will need to come in and have a plaster mould made of his head, and then as soon as we make the mask, we can start at the hospital here.'

'So we will need to be here in Southampton for three months?'

'Yes I'm afraid so: do you have anyone here?'

Lynn said she knew someone who may help and so we discussed the details, as if we were planning a long holiday.

It was decided to tell Peter what was going to happen. Dr Wells was wonderful and explained to him the severity but gave a little hope for some short-term success. Peter seemed to accept the situation: but then he had changed from the man I knew. The vitality had totally gone and in its place was a child-like acceptance.

Dr Wells said he would book us for the months of May to July. It was now the end of March, and we were to return to Sark until Peter was called for a few days in a ward, to prepare him. I had to find somewhere to stay for three months: book a hire car for that time and make arrangements for our cats and home to be looked after: and tell the rest of our families and friends. I was going to need all the strength I could muster. My arrow-prayers were sent quickly and frequently.

3/29

After steroids started to reduce the fluid filling the centre of the tumour and the pressure was lessened, I could almost believe the old Peter was returning. The trip home from Southampton was easy and we talked about the future.

'We need to find somewhere to stay for three months. We can make a holiday of it and drive around to explore the New Forest.' I was not sure if Peter was in denial, or really believed he would be cured: but I played along with it. After all Dr Wells had said we might have another two years.

The month before we were due to return to Southampton was busy with plans. People had to be told. In a place like this tiny island, speculation would be rife and it was easier for the truth to be told. It was hard at first, and it was only with my closest friends I broke down and spoke of the prognosis.

True to her word, Lynn put us in touch with someone who let out a couple of cottages in a village not far from the hospital in Southampton.

'You'll have to change from one to the other a bit, and I'm afraid there are two weeks at the end of June where they are full. Maybe you can find somewhere near the harbour.'

I was relieved to have that problem solved and contacted a car-hire firm we had used before. They gave us a very good rate for three months hire. For a while it was almost like planning a holiday, except Peter usually did the bookings, and now he left it all to me.

The cottages were thatched and well equipped and under any other circumstance I would have enjoyed the lovely location in a friendly village. For the middle two weeks we managed to rent a flat overlooking the Yacht Marina.

We fell into a routine: a lazy morning: a trip to the hospital for Peter's treatment at twelve noon which only took an hour, and then a drive around the country to explore this beautiful part of southern England. It was spring and blossoms showed pink and white in every garden. I renewed my acquaintance with the stately New Forest now bursting with bright green leaves. My family had lived in a suburb of Southampton when my father had been a Customs Officer and we had often taken trips out by bicycle to explore the area.

Now Peter and I toured round by car in the best of English weather, trying to ignore the black cloud which was always hovering nearby. I could almost believe the treatment was working, but realised I was fooling myself. Though slower and more pedantic, Peter appeared almost normal: except for some odd behaviour. I made the mistake of letting him map-read at first, until I realized he was just giving random directions, as a child would. He so wanted to help I let him do several little jobs: one at the end of our stay was to fill up the windscreen-washer water container. It was not until our bill for the hire car was sent, I realized he had topped up the brake fluid container with water, necessitating the whole system to be drained. We were lucky to avoid a serious accident.

I realised then I was on my own and would have to make all the decisions.

For about four months after we returned to Sark, the radiotherapy appeared to have helped. I was instructed to juggle the steroids, depending on Peter's condition, but they had the effect of causing Peter to put on so much weight that he looked like a benign Buddha.

We tried to live as normal a life as we could, but gradually we had to resort to a wheelchair. For the first time I regretted the absence of cars on Sark. It would have been so much easier to drive around instead of having to push a wheelchair over stony roads.

I tried to take Peter to as many things as we could together: church: friends' houses: public occasions like the church fete, and even to have a meal at our favourite hotel. The owners, who were friends, suggested we use a convenient ground-floor room and stay overnight.

Once or twice we went over to Guernsey, as I tried to keep my clinic going, having held phone consultations while we were in Southampton. It was impossible for Peter to walk around, but we managed occasionally. I had made friends with an Austrian owner of a pleasant cafe, visiting in the past several times to enjoy her traditional apple strudel. She kindly kept an eye on Peter while I managed to see a few patients, but gradually it became more difficult. Eventually I arranged for a friend to stay as a companion in Sark while I went on my own to the neighbouring island. Peter was not happy about that. His possessiveness had increased with his dependence and after one unpleasant occasion, I had to abandon my trips.

When I returned from this clinic, I discovered the friend fast asleep in the lounge. Peter was not with him and so I went to the bedroom. I knew he could walk around the house by supporting himself on the walls but was not prepared for what I discovered. He was lying half in and half out of the bathroom, with no lower garments: the bathroom was awash with urine. As I ran towards him I noticed there was a pillow from the bed under Peter's head. It was only later I realised it could not have been put there by our babysitting friend.

'Are you alright my darling? I'll not leave you again.'

'No, you'd better not. I might hurt myself next time.'

I knew I was being manipulated, but I also knew we did not have much more time together and it was a small price to pay.

The falls became frequent, and I was fortunate to be able to buy a mechanical seat. It was mainly for use in a bath, but I could get Peter to wriggle onto it and pump it up until he could stand again.

We had a spa bath installed when we rebuilt the cottage, and Peter loved to be lowered into it, however it became difficult to get him out. One time he got in, being lowered by the mechanical seat, but he then slipped off and I just could not get him to wriggle back onto it to winch him out. I realised I would have to get in with Peter, to help him so I stripped off and we managed together. As I was drying him, a flash of the old Peter showed as he chuckled, 'Not many nurses would get in the bath with their patients!'

The times were few and far between I would see my dear friend and lover again. The strain was sometimes too much, and I had to let off the steam of frustration. Once when I was in the kitchen, I could feel it boiling up and let out a scream and yelled; 'I can't stand it!'

A little later when I was with Peter he said; 'What was that noise I heard?'

'Oh, er, I trod on the cat's tail.'

Most of the time, I had to accept the tumour had made Peter return to a dependant childhood. It made me sympathise with people who looked after sufferers of Alzheimer's dementia.

We managed to get out and about on fine days, using the wheelchair. There were sometimes a few problems when we were in public if he wanted to go to the toilet, as happened in church one Sunday. He would just start to pull his trousers down, and I had to act quickly. I became adept at getting him onto the wheelchair and to the nearest 'Gents', just hoping no-one else came in.

Night-time was a problem too, as Peter seemed unable to turn over. As a district nurse, I had learned to fold a sheet in half across the bed, under the patient, leaving a length at one side of the bed: it was then quite easy to cross one of the patient's ankles over the other and pull the sheet through with the patient on it, and flip him over. I was worried about bedsores and had to do this several times a night: I did not get much sleep until I hired mechanical assistance.

When I was a district nurse looking after terminal patients, I had often been surprised the partner of the very ill patient still slept in the same double bed. I now realised how important that is for both people. However ill a person is, contact is vital, and I now know from my experience comfort and strength can come from it.

3/30

The months passed and December approached. We were to return to the Southampton hospital to be assessed early in that month. My 60th birthday was due on the first of December, but I had not expected any celebrations. Still showing a few surprises, Peter suddenly announced.

'I would like to give you a big party for your birthday, and I want you to go to Guernsey and buy a nice party frock.' He shakily wrote a generous cheque as I tried to hide my tears.

How I still loved this guy.

The trip to Guernsey was a treat, and friends looked after Peter for the day. I chose a lovely silky suit with snug-fitting jacket, long skirt and trousers to match in a gold colour. I even had time to see a few patients at my clinic.

When I dressed up to show Peter he seemed a little disappointed.

'I thought you would get a nice frilly frock...but if you like it...'

We invited about 30 friends to our favourite hotel, and they put on a wonderful buffet, and we stayed the night. Both my brother David from Holland and Roy from Sweden came over too, which was wonderful. It was a bitter-sweet occasion, as we all knew it would probably be a 'good-bye' party for Peter too, but he raised himself for the occasion. I never really knew if he realised how ill he was: if the apparent return to childhood was genuine, or a defence against reality.

Peter's daughter Lynn and family had moved to a new house in a converted chapel in England and Peter said he wanted to go there for Christmas. I was not sure if he was well enough but was pleased he showed some interest. We agreed we would return to Sark after his hospital appointment and then go up to Lynn a few days before the holiday.

It was not to work out like that.

After the party Peter seemed more confused, and it was with difficulty we managed to reach Southampton. I had to arrange to have a carry-on seat to get him down the steep steps at the Sark harbour, and the boat crew were wonderful in steering to a ramp in Guernsey where the taxi could get to the water's edge. I took a wheelchair with me, and we made the rest of the journey with considerable help from the airline staff.

We had some wonderful friends who lived in Southampton and they insisted we stay while attending the follow-up appointment. I shall never forget the generosity and selflessness of my friend. Some time after our stay she confided in me she had a diagnosis of breast cancer while we were staying with her. She said nothing to me at the time, but later told me my problems took the worry from her concern about herself.

I knew Peter was getting worse and my fear the tumour had grown again were confirmed by Dr Wells after he had made his examination. He took us both into his office and gave us the bad news.

'I am sorry, Mr Curtis, there is nothing else we can do.'

'You can operate again: give some more radiotherapy? There must be something!' For the first time Peter was shaken from his apparent acceptance. I realised then he really had convinced himself he might get better.

From that moment Peter's fight went and he seemed to have no interest in anything. I decided it would be best to go straight to his daughter, rather than both go back to Sark first as planned.

'The doctor said you can stay in the hospital a few days and they will sort out your steroids. I will go back to Sark and get all the Christmas presents and collect you. Then we'll go up to Lynn's. OK?'

I was not sure if Peter had understood, and it was with a heavy heart I returned to Sark. The weather turned wild, and the boats were cancelled for a couple of days. It was a week before I returned to the Hospital.

What I found broke my heart.

'Mr Curtis seemed to think you had left him here. He has been so difficult. Won't eat, and we had to put a catheter in as he was wetting the bed.'

My poor Peter was in quite a state, and it took me hours to convince him he had not been abandoned. I realised he was in no shape to do other than return to Sark with me.

'You'll never manage on your own.' The nurses were concerned, trying to persuade me to keep Peter hospitalised.

'Of course I will: it is what I have been doing for years. It's a poor thing if I can't do it for the man I love.'

I phoned the St John ambulance equipment loan department in Guernsey, whom I had used on many occasions in the past and I tried to be business-like. I could not cope with sympathy at this time as there was too much to organise.

'I need a hoist; hospital bed; commode and a ripple mattress, please.' I gave my address and was relieved they could all be delivered a day before we would return to Sark. I was not sure how I would get everything set up, but I decided to think about that later. In the meantime, I had to arrange an ambulance from the hospital to the Southampton airport: an ambulance from Guernsey airport to the Sark boat: help to carry Peter onto the boat and the Sark ambulance at the other end. He had deteriorated so much all this was now necessary. I decided to ask my friends on the Sark Ambulance to help me set everything up, but in the event it was not necessary.

Everything went like clockwork. The ambulance people were wonderful, driving right to the plane and carrying Peter on and off by a carry-seat.

I had phoned David and Hilly to tell them we were returning, and what had happened. Bless them, they had assembled all the equipment: put the heating on and even put a vase of flowers in our bedroom for when we arrived.

We had a quiet Christmas. I had nothing in the house, having planned to be with Lynn, but David and Hilly brought food over.

Whether it was the advancing tumour, or the fact Peter had given up, the end came quite quickly. My days were taken up with what we nurses used to call 'heavy nursing.' Everything had to be done for Peter, from shaving, feeding, washing and the more intimate personal things. The ripple mattress, like the one I had used for Hap, helped to prevent bedsores. Thanks to the hoist I was able to get Peter up and into the lounge most days and I blessed the advice we had been given to have wider passageways when planning the re- building.

The family visited regularly, as did our friends, and I was able to pop out for a walk or a coffee occasionally. Towards the middle of January 2001 I had made a plan to have lunch with a friend while two others were coming in to sit with Peter. He had stopped eating anything but ice-cream and jelly and I knew he was slipping into a coma, but I used to put the radio on his pillow as I was sure he could hear it. On this day, an hour or so before I was due to go out, I tuned into the music programme and bent over to kiss Peter's forehead: his eyebrows flicked and there was a faint smile on his lips.

A moment later I heard the programme change to talking and went in to alter it. I looked at Peter and realised he had slipped away.

The reaction did not set in immediately. I phoned the doctor, and the mechanism was put into motion which I had so often done before for others.

It was the end of an era, but somehow I had to go on living.

There was so much to attend to for the next few weeks I did not have much time for grief.

The tears came later.

There was a funeral to arrange, and a cremation and wake in Guernsey for immediate friends and family. We decided we should have a proper send-off in April, when relatives and friends from overseas could attend. In the event it was the sort of occasion Peter would have loved: a well-known cellist performed in the church in a lively service. People were asked to wear bright clothes, and a large party for 200 guests was held in the hall.

Later I and the family went to Peter's favourite beach of Grande Greve to scatter his ashes. Even that had a lighter note as the wind flurried and sent his ashes scuttling, so we had to dodge to avoid getting covered with them.

It was then time for me to decide what to do with the rest of my life. I did not want to stay where Peter and I had been so happy; there were too many memories. I sold Le Clos des Camps and bought the derelict old place I used to visit called 'Le Hurel,' it seemed a lifetime ago. It was just the sort of challenge I needed to keep me sane and stop me wallowing in unremitting grief. It needed a great deal of renovation, and I threw myself into decorating and basic joinery, often working through the night. Then I turned to the garden which had been left like a builders' yard, creating a beautiful cottage garden. It was even featured on a local television show.

Gradually my life settled to a level of normality, but my loss was to haunt me for the rest of my life. I began to be grateful for the happiness I had for seventeen years, instead of regretting those years I would never have.

My clinics in Guernsey and nursing on Sark grew and I used an extension wing in the cottage to offer self-catering, but in the back of my mind was the thought of returning to New Zealand, where my son Roy and family had returned from Sweden.

For several years I hesitated, travelling over each of my winters to see Roy.

Then came the financial crash in the UK and my investments which were my main source of income, dried up.

I had to make another major decision.

✼✼✼✼✼✼✼✼✼✼✼✼

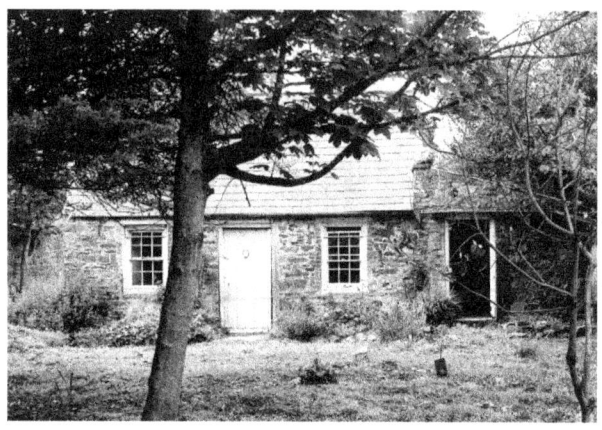

Le Hurel before renovation

It was time to leave Sark, so in 2009 I packed my personal belongings in many boxes, sold my little cottage and most of the furniture and emigrated once more, back to New Zealand, to begin yet another phase of my life.

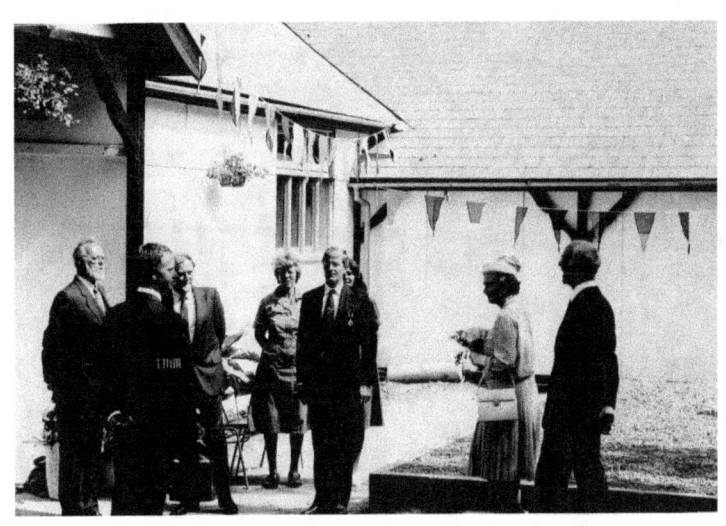

The visit of Queen Elizabeth and Prince Phillip

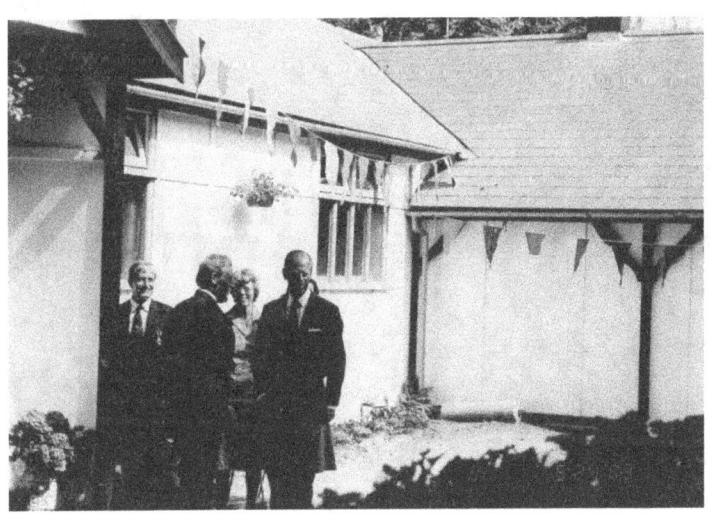

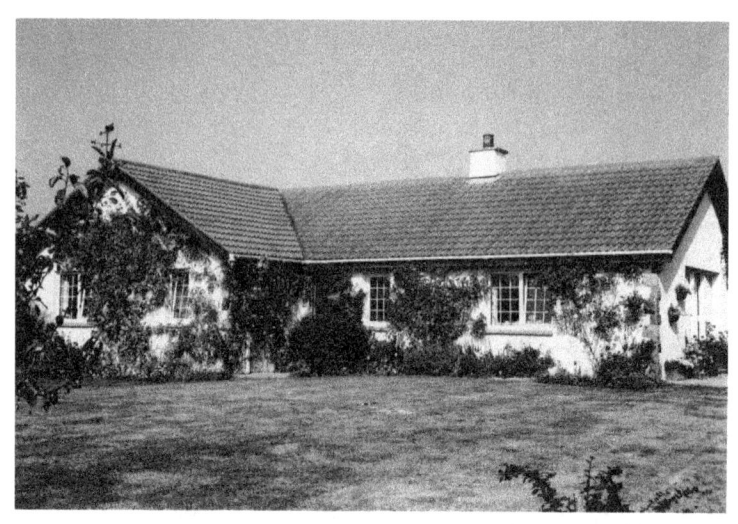

Rebuild of Le Clos des Camps

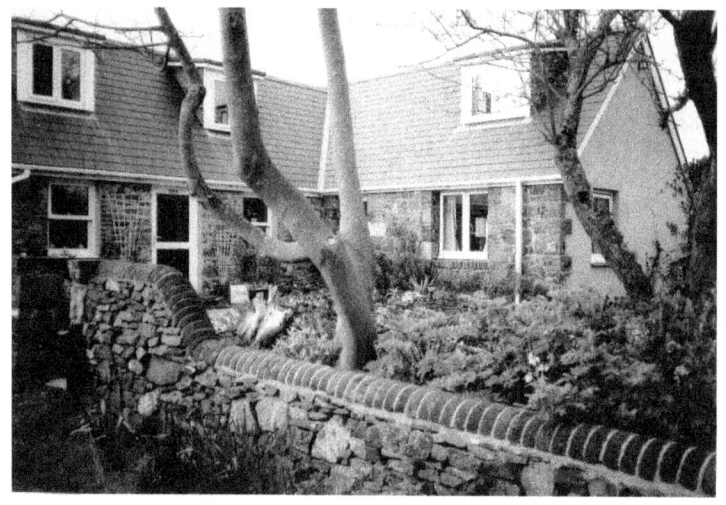

Rebuild of Le Hurel

PART 4
NEW ZEALAND
1972-1974 and 1976-1984
2009---?

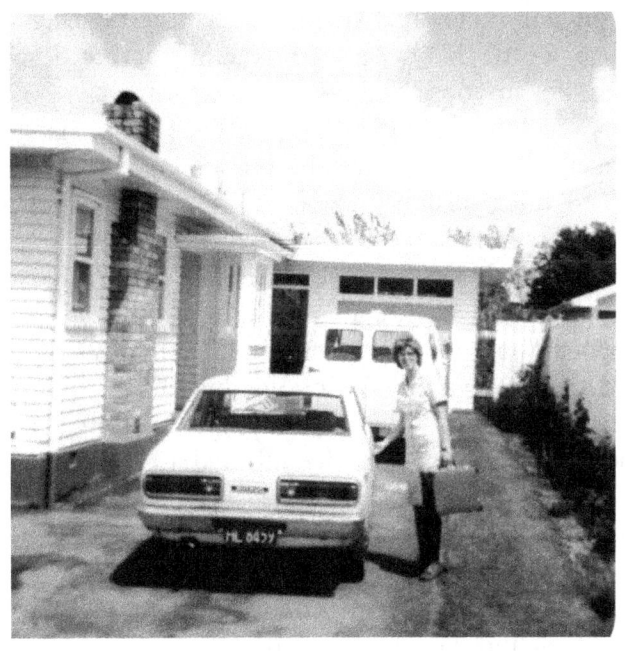

Chris as N Z District Nurse

4/1

After leaving Sark in 1972 for our two-year tour of New Zealand I was not sure if I would have the chance to nurse there, but I took the precaution of registering with the appropriate authorities. It was not enough to hold the UK practicing certificate.

To my amazement my first application was turned down, until I realised some of the wording on the form was unclear regarding hours spent in theoretical training, just mentioning lectures. It did not include tutorials and ward instruction, and so it appeared the applicant did not have enough theoretical study. Not willing to accept this, I wrote to the New Zealand Nursing authorities; was thanked for my observations, and the form was rewritten. I was secretly proud I had effected a change in bureaucracy but had to wonder how many applicants had accepted the decision and not been able to practice in New Zealand in the past.

Our extensive trip out by ship was very enjoyable; although it was so rough most of the time I was in a permanent state of queasiness, until a fellow passenger introduced me to a mix of port and brandy, taken in small sips. It certainly settled that horrible empty 'I have nothing left to bring up,' feeling and I could enjoy the excellent food. It was an Italian ship and as Ken and I loved cuisine from that country, we were in our element.

I also admired the handsome waiters and crew; and was secretly flattered when one of the young men who served the children's meals, tried to date me.

Eventually we arrived in Auckland, the largest city in the country, and were met by a friend we had known in Sark. She had booked us into a motel for a week and then it became decision time. We had to get driving licenses as neither of us had needed one before. Ken had never driven, but I had been having lessons on and off for years. My father started to instruct me on his huge Daimler...his hobby and, pride and joy...but it was a heavy car and I never bothered to take lessons, as first I went for my training and then of course we had not owned one on the car-free island of Sark.

'We need to find somewhere to live while we search for a van and learn to drive the thing, and of course equip it for our new life.'

'And get jobs until we are ready to go. It is late summer now...funny to think of February as summer...so we need to be ready, say in October.' Ken had been studying a New Zealand calendar; 'There's a public holiday called *'Labour Day'* late in that month; whatever that is, so what say we aim to set off just after that?'

Within a few days I had managed to have an interview in a small private hospital in one of Auckland's leafy suburbs. The advertisement in the paper had said a sister-in-charge was needed for medical and post operative patients. When I met the owner Matron, she had a different story to tell after she had discussed the details of my nursing experience and my current situation.

'Actually Mrs Davies, what I really need is a resident acting Matron. I have been told by my doctor to have a rest...a heart problem...but I dare not mention accommodation was included or I would be inundated with applicants; it is so difficult to find inexpensive places here.' For a moment Mrs Mason looked at me, then obviously came to a decision.

'You say you can only offer about eight months, but that should be long enough. I would first like to meet your husband and son...I'm not sure a three-year-old would be suitable in that flat; it has some nice furniture...' I was about to retort, but held my tongue as I was pretty sure when she met Roy he would win her over. He was a quiet, sweet natured lad, keen on his Lego and small jigsaws and not likely to be a noisy tearaway. After all he had grown up in a guest house among people all his life and had learned if not 'to be seen and not heard,' at least to be un-demanding. We arranged for Ken and Roy to accompany me the next day to meet Mrs Mason, and by the following week we moved into the delightful small flat above the main part of the hospital. The only disadvantage was that there was only one bedroom, but Mrs Mason lent us a camp bed and Roy had his little area screened off in a corner of the large lounge.

Monday came too quickly, and I found it difficult to adjust to nursing again. I had not worked in a hospital for several years, and although this was only a small private one, there were staff to contend with and medical routines to adhere to.

Mrs Mason was waiting in the office as I walked down from the flat. I had been given a white dress and cap so at least I felt the part.

'Now, I think you should meet the staff. You have a nurse aid on duty this morning, Hoki Patu. She is Maori and very efficient, and you also have Bella Priest,' she said as we walked towards the kitchen. 'Well, she will be a good nurse one day I expect, when she stops chasing everything in trousers.' She pushed the door open into the kitchen and I was met by a pair of baleful eyes glaring at me from a red-faced woman standing by a large cooker. 'And this is Betty Tuff, our cook.' I was about to say 'Hello' but was forestalled by the cook's comment.

'So, this is the new *'Pom'* in charge of us all is it?' She glowered at me. 'Well, if you keep out of my kitchen and don't interfere, we will get on. Tuff by name and tough by nature, that's me. Now get out of my kitchen, I have breakfast to cook.'

I looked at Mrs Mason and expected some reprimand, but was surprised to see her smiling. 'All right Betty, I am sure you two will get on.'

As we walked out and along the corridor, she explained 'I have known Betty Tuff for many years. She has a heart of gold really. She was cook at a huge sheep station in Australia for years, and she still thinks she has *jackaroos* to organise.' She stopped by the drug room.

'You will be OK if you do what she says.'

'Like heck' I thought. 'I am not going to be bossed around like that. I know she will have a weak spot and I just needed to find it.'

The day wore on and developed a pattern. It was a little like riding a bicycle. Once you had done it, familiarity took over, and the hospital routine soon fell into place. Cups of tea and meals for the patients, washes, baths and bed baths, drug rounds, dressings, special treatments, toilet rounds and doctors' visits.

'Each patient has his or her own doctor, of course,' Mrs Mason had explained, 'as they are private patients.'

I was unprepared for the first visit from a New Zealand doctor. I was reading some of the patients' notes when a shadow in the doorway cut out the light.

'I would like to see Tom Banks, nurse.' I looked up to see an attractive man leaning on the door frame. He had on an open necked shirt, shorts and knee-length socks, the standard uniform of New Zealand men.

'Sorry, I said in my best 'Matron's' voice,', 'visiting is over until this evening. Maybe you could come back then?'

'You're new, aren't you? Well, I had better introduce myself. I am Dr Ian Carter, and I am a bit too busy to come back tonight.'

I leapt up blushing, scattering the case notes all over the floor. 'Well, you should look like a doctor. Where's your white coat?' The comment slipped out before I could stop it. 'Sorry, I mean, er, I'll take you to him...'

'No need nurse, I know my way.' And he winked at me.

Certainly, things were much more casual in this country.

4/2

By the second week I was beginning to enjoy myself and the staff seemed to know the routine well. I had been in charge of 30-bed wards with a staff of several nurses in the past and soon discovered the strengths and weaknesses of my new nurses. But I still ran afoul of Mrs *'Tuff-by-name-and-tough-by-nature'*.

It was at the beginning of the second week when my phone rang as I was dressing to go on duty. I could hardly hear the voice at the other end ... 'not well, got a headache: s'bad.'

I realised it was the slurred voice of my cook. If I had not thought I knew better I would have suspected` she was the worse for drink.

'Well, er, that's OK. Come in when you can.'

'You'll have to arrange a relief cook.'

'Yes. Well don't you worry.' I stood a moment staring at the phone as I put down the receiver, then made a decision. I had run a guest house for seven years; surely I could cook a few meals for patients.

The menus were all written on a board in the kitchen, so it was easy to plan meals.

'Right,' I told my nurses. 'Mrs T is not well today.' I saw the exchange of looks which confirmed my suspicions. 'So, we will have to cope on our own.' And cope we did. Everyone did their bit, and I managed to cook the meals between drug rounds and doctor's visits. I left the evening meal ready to be served and finally staggered up the steps to the flat much later than usual.

'I was beginning to worry. I thought I should start supper,' was all Ken said, and I was grateful not to have the job of cooking our own evening meal

'Well, it has been a day and a half, but now I know how to cope with Mrs T.'

The next morning as I saw the cook enter the main door, I called her in to the office. 'Are you better? I hope you don't mind, but I did the cooking myself. Your menus are excellent and what a tidy kitchen you have.' Betty Tuff opened her mouth to make some comment, but I continued, 'if you should have a recurrence of your ... er ... headache, I think we can cope. I used to have my own guest house, you know. I would love to see how you make that lovely seameal custard pudding though; mine did not set properly.'

'Yes well, I'll do it for tea today, if you really want to know.' She looked me in the eye. 'You're not bad, for a *'Pom'.*'

It was a new experience for me to be in sole charge of a small hospital. For the first few weeks Mrs Mason came in to see how I was managing, but her health was clearly not good and more and more I was left to manage on my own.

I was the only fully qualified nurse, although two of the staff were trained nurse aids. That meant they could do basic nursing but could not put out medicines or make decisions on treatments. I was supposed to attend to all the needs of the various doctors who called to see their patients; prepare the rosters for the nurses; arrange treatments; talk to relatives; order medical and domestic supplies before they ran out; supervise cleaning staff and find replacements for those who did not turn up for work. I stood in for the cook, when she had one of her 'headaches', and sometimes found myself dusting and cleaning when one of the domestic staff failed to turn up for duty.

I was also on call for any emergencies 24 hours a day. Problems seemed to occur mostly at night. There was a nurse-aid on then, but she had to ring me on the internal phone if there were any situations she could not handle. Often this would be the death of one of the post-hip-fracture patients. It happened in about 40% of these ladies. So much so, I used to take the relatives to one side after admission and explain about post operative shock. I felt it did not look very good on the hospital records, to have such a mortality rate.

Although there were many of these patients, there were also longer-term ones such as Tom Banks, slowly dying of cancer. He was a delightful, elderly man. A real gentleman and I used to love to stop and chat with him when I had time. He had been a heavy smoker and knew he had only himself to blame for his lung cancer. 'But Chris,' he used to wheeze, 'what's the point in life, if you can't indulge your vices?' The twinkle in his eye made me realise smoking had not been the only 'vice' he had indulged.

Quite a different story was Dorothy Pugh. She had had a severe stroke but eventually recovered most of her movement. It was her character which had been affected more severely. I read in her notes she was a respectable retired teacher: a spinster and pillar of her church. She was a large woman, now almost uncontrollable unless sedated, and the language issuing from her prim mouth made even my hair curl. I could not but wonder where she had heard many of the words, or if she even understood them.

One night the internal flat phone rang by our bed.

'So sorry, Sister, but I have lost Miss Pugh.'

'What do you mean, lost her?'

'Well, I went in to check her, and she wasn't there. She couldn't have gone out of the main door as it is locked of course, and I have looked everywhere.'

'OK I'll be down.' I told the sleepy Ken what had happened as I leapt out of bed.

As I ran down the stairs in my nightdress and dressing gown, I realised the window at the side of the stairway was open and I could see out onto the top of the carport. I glimpsed a flash of white nightdress and stopped horrified while I watched my missing patient slide off the roof and start to walk down the drive to the road.

'Quick, get me the drug keys. She's legging it up the road. I may have to give her a shot of *Largactile*, or I'll never get her back,' I gasped as the nurse appeared.

Suitably armed I bolted out of the door and ran up the quiet road clad only in my night clothes. Miss Pugh was just ahead and was obviously tiring.

I caught up with her just before she made the main road. 'Miss Pugh, Miss Pugh, where are you going at this time of night, and with only your nighty on?'

She turned and glowered at me. Made some profane remark and started to hit me on the head with her handbag.

'Right, well I did try,' I gulped as I stuck the needle through the thin nightdress. The drug took a little while to act, but I tried to talk soothingly, and then wondered how I would get her back to the hospital as she suddenly sat down on the pavement with a thud.

The cavalry arrived in the form of Ken pushing a wheelchair. My night nurse had alerted him.

'Am I glad to see you.'

Ken shook his head with a grin, 'Never a dull moment, being married to you.'

4/3

The months of work and preparation passed quickly. Ken obtained a rather boring job in Woolworths warehouse, but within a short while was promoted to junior management. Roy spent some time in a nearby day care centre, and enjoyed playing with his little friends, while I learned all about the interesting and very different country we planned to explore for two years. I was not sure if I would be nursing again during our travels but was content to take whatever job came my way.

Both having passed New Zealand driving tests, we bought a large white Bedford van. It was just a basic delivery vehicle and we equipped it as best we could, but there was no luxury.

As time passed we felt less like 'new-chums'. I had anticipated New Zealand would be different from England and it was, but in some strange, unexpected ways. Our friend Mary and the hospital staff were a great help in my understanding some of the peculiarities, but I learned others the hard way.

One I found particularly amusing was the telephone. Once, I was dialling a phone number without looking what I was doing. It was totally wrong, and I realised the numbers were the opposite way round. The '9' was at the top and the '1' and '0' at the bottom of the dial, whereas in UK it was the reverse. The emergency call was '111' instead of what I was used to, '999'.

On another occasion, I was chatting to the nurses on a tea break (or 'smoko' as they called it), and I said, 'we are making progress with the van, we are just going to convert it ...' and they all started laughing.

'You don't want to say that,' exclaimed Hoki. 'That means you stole it!

Another expression which amused me was the way my staff usually said *"hooray"* as they left to go home. At first I thought they must be relieved to be off duty, until I realised it was just their way of saying 'goodbye'.

There was also the way many people answered the phone with, 'are you there?' I had to refrain from a suitable retort.

After my first meeting with Dr Carter I became used to the casual dress and manner of the medical staff and New Zealand people generally. It was quite common to see even the older schoolboys walking about in shorts and with bare feet, but with the regulation ties and shirts. I heard the story of a schoolmaster arriving from the UK to take up a post in a local secondary school. When he saw the tough, hairy-legged pupils walking to school in bare feet, he turned right back and left the country. An exaggeration I felt, but there was something primitive and virile about the casual dress and manner of New Zealand men which made the pioneer days seem recent. The whole city of Auckland, and I suspected New Zealand, was bursting with vigour and vitality. The traffic was more aggressive, the vegetation invasive, the flowers brilliant and the population bustling with activity. It seemed to declare. *'We are a new country, and we are going somewhere in this tired old world.'*

Eventually it was time to say 'goodbye' to Mrs Mason, the staff and patients in the hospital, and part of me was quite sad. It had been a challenge and a new experience for me and had encouraged confidence in myself. After seven years with only a few patients to look after in a totally different and un-clinical situation, I was relieved to realise I was still able to cope as a nurse.

For the next four months Ken, Roy and I toured all over New Zealand, mostly living in the van, visiting camp sites when we needed hot showers and to stock up on home baking. Just before Christmas in 1972, we needed to top up our finances so were lucky enough to be employed by a motel owner in a small village called Renwick, neat Blenheim in the South Island. The attraction for us was that the owners, Rich and Connie, owned several horses and carriages. We both had learned to drive on Sark and look after horses and carriages, and so we were able to take the motel clients for carriage trips. This was rather different from our other jobs in New Zealand but a couple of times my nursing experience came in handy.

The first time was not long after we arrived. Ken was set to work looking after the horses. There was not enough grass, and he often had to take them out to graze on the riverbanks. The fields Rich used were badly fenced, and one day a horse called King tried to jump the fence and a thin piece of broken fencing threaded through a small part of his buttock, like a stitch, holding him fast.

'You're a nurse, Chris, can't you cut it out?' King, was starting to panic and something had to be done. I had some basic surgical instruments in my first aid box which I had brought with me from Sark, not knowing what to expect in our travels. Among them was a scalpel so I approached the horse with the knife clasped in my hand, standing well to the side in case he lashed out with his hooves. As the piece of fence was wedged tightly, the skin and flesh were taught. With memories of my days in the minor ops department in Whittington hospital in London I slashed deeply, cutting down to the wood of the fence and King jumped free. I stepped quickly to the side, while the men soothed the frightened animal holding a dressing to the cut. The vet was called after the horse was taken to his stable.

The wound was cleaned, stitched, and dusted with antibiotics and as he packed his bag, the vet grinned at me; 'You did a good job there, though a bit unorthodox.'

The second time involved Rich's daughter Maggie who lived quite near, married to a farm manager. She was expecting her first child, and everyone was excited as the weeks passed. We spent our first Charismas in New Zealand with the family, and it was so strange to be eating hot food outside in the middle of summer, especially as it was about 30 degrees in the shade.

Rich gave us a week off so we packed up to tour further south, enjoying the freedom once more, but agreed to return for the busy school holidays in January. As we were driving back into the motel entrance the house door flew open and Connie ran out, 'thank goodness you're here. Quick Chris, it's Maggie; she's bleeding. I think it's the baby.'

I jumped out almost before the van stopped and rushed into the house. Maggie was sitting on the settee with legs splayed and I could see blood seeping through her clothes, and she was crying. 'Oh, Chris, it's too early, I'm only seven months.'

I took charge.

'Right: got to get you to hospital straight away. Connie, lie Maggie down as flat as you can. Head down and pack pillows under her bottom and legs to lift them up; and pad some towels between her legs.' I called Ken in. 'We need to get Maggie to hospital, OK if we take her in the van? It will be quicker than waiting for an ambulance. Rich, could you call the Hospital and let them know we are on the way?' The men made a makeshift stretcher from blankets, and we rolled our mattresses out on the floor of the van for Maggie to lie on. Ken drove slowly to the Hospital; Connie stayed with her daughter while the rest of us returned wearily home. We all felt unsettled, and I was glad we had bought a lobster on our way home as we did not feel like cooking. Maggie's husband Matthew was away fishing with some friends and Maggie had been staying with her parents.

We returned to the van to sleep and were awoken early next morning by Rich banging on the door. 'She's going to be alright; and the baby, thank goodness. They say your quick action probably saved it. Can't thank you enough,' he said gruffly. 'She insisted on doing some cleaning for us, silly girl, and must have done too much. She's got to take it easy for a while.

As soon as the school holidays were over, off we drove again, covering the rest of the beautiful South Island, but winter was approaching again and we decided to return to Auckland. I contacted Mrs Mason and was delighted to be taken on again in my old position. Mrs Tuff just nodded to me as I peeped in the kitchen, even admitting I was an improvement on the agency nurses who had been working there over the summer.

For the winter we carried on as before and then set off for our final tour, heading first up to the far north of the North Island. All too soon our two years of wandering came to an end, but we had fallen in love with the lovely country.

'What would you think of investigating returning here, Chris?' Ken's question was no real surprise to me.

'What about Sark?'

'Do you really want to carry on with running a guest house? And I would like to maybe have a proper apiary; wonderful opportunity. Then there is Roy to think of. Schooling is excellent here and he would have a good life.'

'And maybe I could be a district nurse here...'

'That might be possible, but you should discover what qualifications you need. It may not be the same as England.'

For the last few weeks in New Zealand we investigated the possibility, and I discovered I would have to take a midwifery course to be a registered maternity nurse/district nurse in New Zealand.

Our property in Sark was rented out for three years, allowing me time to take the shortened midwifery course in London.

4/4

After the six-month midwifery course and a return to Sark to keep the business running for the summer, we advertised for someone to buy a lease for ten years. We decided not to sell outright as insurance in case things did not work out in New Zealand. A decision which I was to be very grateful for in the future.

Again Ken's advertising experience came in very handy, as we had many applications although I did wonder about a few replies such as...'I have always wanted to live in the Scottish Islands.'

Eventually we picked on a young couple from Jersey who were expecting their first baby. We reasoned they would at least know what island life was like and sold them a ten-year lease for enough to allow us to buy a house and a car or another van in New Zealand. At that time the exchange rate was in our favour and property was cheap in New Zealand.

We packed a couple of suitcases each, arranging to have most of our belongings sent out by freighter. We were travelling on a Greek ship this time, and passing through the Suez Canal, as it was newly opened after the previous troubles in that part of the world. It was nowhere as good as the Italian line and started badly from the first day. The sailing instructions informed us the clothes needed for the trip were sent to a 'baggage room' to be collected once the ship set sail. A small case each was all we were allowed in the cabin on embarkation. All other baggage went down in the hold until we arrived in Auckland. After we had left England Ken went down to collect our travel cases, but they were nowhere to be found.

We went to see the head steward who looked at the manifest.

'I am sorry, Mr and Mrs Davies...all your cases were sent down to the hold.'

'But we only have a change of clothes; can't you get them back?'

'Sorry.'

Poor Roy only had a pair of long thick trousers and the ship's shop had no clothes for a six-year-old boy. I was relieved I had packed one long skirt and top and was able to buy another blouse and a swimming costume. Ken seldom wore shorts anyway and bought a couple of shirts. In the end I cut Roy's trousers to make a pair of shorts. Later in our shore trips we purchased more exotic clothes, which possibly we would not have done otherwise.

We arrived once more in New Zealand, but this time our thoughts were centred round finding a house and getting work. For a while I toyed with the idea of contacting Mrs Mason again, but decided I wanted to be a rural district nurse as soon as possible.

It was not going to be so easy.

I applied to the district nursing headquarters, but there was nothing available.

'You are well qualified, Mrs Davies, but rural postings don't come up that often in the Auckland area...now if you'd like to look at the South Island, or up in the Far North...?'

We had decided to stay in or near Auckland; the few friends we had made lived there, and we both loved the sub-tropical weather and the lifestyle. I put my name on the waiting list and looked for another nursing job in the meantime.

'We'll buy something to live in, until you get a post you like,' Ken agreed. It was not long before we found a suitable house in a suburb called Mount Roskill. It was a typical weatherboard-clad building with corrugated iron roof. Lawns surrounded the white-painted bungalow, and a small deck opened from the front. Exotic lemon, orange and grapefruit trees grew there, and there were several flowering shrubs scattered throughout the garden. It was in good condition, although the interior decor would not have been our choice with flower-patterned wallpaper and carpets.

'It'll do for the moment,' we decided.

Ken got a job back in the Woolworths' warehouse and soon his ability and obvious intelligence earned him promotion to a junior managerial post again. In the meantime, I needed a job which enabled me to be home with Roy when Ken was at work as we had enrolled Roy in a nearby school. As nurses are needed 24 hours a day, I soon landed a position in a large retirement village.

My duties were to look after 300 elderly residents housed in accommodation ranging from independent cottages, through communal houses and en-suite rooms to two hospital wards. I started at 4pm and finished any time after 11pm.

I was the only registered nurse on duty, and my staff were mostly untrained care assistants who had come straight from the Cook or Samoan Islands. I learned the hard way they had not a clue about nursing procedures.

Soon after starting the job, I was on one of the hospital wards where the less-well elderly were sent from their other accommodation to be looked after. Distracted by the myriad of things I had to remember, I asked one of the nurses to take a bedpan to a particular lady, as I whisked down the ward.

A few minutes later, I walked back up the ward and saw the nurse holding the bedpan beside the patient's bed, but not making any effort to put the poor lady on it.

'What's the matter nurse?' I asked, a little irritated.

'Please miss, I don't know how to do it.'

I realised then I would have to start from 'square one'. In fact, when instructed properly, the girls made very good nurses. It was in their culture to look after and care for the elderly and nothing was too much trouble for them.

In the meantime, I had to accustom myself to administering medication and care to many residents who hardly knew the time of day let alone their names. After a few unsuccessful occasions when I called out someone's name and several people answered, I hit on the idea of delegating a few of the more alert residents to aid me until I knew everyone.

The job left me my days free, although after I had seen Roy off to school, I was sometimes so tired I went back to bed. Soon I became more accustomed to my hours, and I started to look after our garden and enjoyed mowing the lawn with our new petrol mower. Memories of Sark came back to me, but this was a really good mower and I enjoyed the exercise.

One day a neighbour stopped me while I was finishing off the front lawn.

'I've often seen you doing that; you wouldn't come and do ours would you? My Bill has a wonky heart, and I can't cope with the garden.'

'OK, if you like.' And so I began a lawn mowing round in my spare time. Ken caught the bus to work, so I had the use of the new van we had bought, during the day, which fitted in well. I loved to be outdoors, and the smell of the cut grass and exotic flowers made me feel I was in the country, instead of the centre of the largest city in New Zealand.

4/5

At last I saw an advertisement for a rural district nursing job in an area we both liked. It was just north of the city, on the east coast, with a beautiful beach. Full of excitement, I rang the district nursing supervisor with my hopes.

'I am sorry, Christine, I am not sure it is quite what you are looking for. I think you need a more rural setting.' My heart sank as I had set my sights on this job, but she continued, 'I should not really say this yet, and it will have to be advertised, but I think there is an area coming up soon that will really suit you. It has a house and car included but it is a 24 hour call position.'

'Well, that would not be a worry.' After all, I had just spent seven years on 24-hour call running a guest house and doubling as a nurse on Sark.

I attended an interview and was accepted as sole rural nurse in an area with eight villages and a diameter of over 30 miles. Most of the roads were unsealed gravel and the population was a mix of Chinese market gardeners, Dalmatian vintners, Māori, established farmers, retired country people, and 'alternative-life stylers'. I was under the supervision of a central 'Extramural Hospital' and directly responsible to the western region unit.

Otherwise, I was on my own.

It was a far cry from my London days. In this new job, I was sent notification of patients directly from a doctor, a hospital or from my immediate superiors. In most cases I had to decide how often a patient needed visiting and fit them into my day as best I could. Sometimes it was a daily visit; as for diabetics requiring insulin injections or someone needing dressings. On other occasions it may be only once a week; but more often, two or three times a day and into the night, if it was a terminal case. As well as this, I held clinics at my rooms if a patient could get to me, and of course there were emergencies, which often seemed to happen in the middle of the night. Thank goodness I was not practicing as a midwife, although I did have to visit mums and their newly delivered babies. I always made myself available by phone, and this was seldom abused, with people only contacting me if they were really worried.

It was hard work, but I loved the freedom. I was almost my own boss, as I was soon left to cope when I had proved myself competent. Sure, I was often up in the night, but could fit my hours round family commitments and be there for Roy when needed.

Ken soon found work in the many orchards and eventually became an apiarist, which he had said he wanted to be. He took his hives from orchard to orchard to help with pollination. The hives we had on Sark had trained Ken and now he became an expert at bee management, eventually having ten hives. My more mercurial temperament was not compatible with beekeeping; especially when I became allergic to bee venom. I discovered this dramatically when one day I was with Ken in the van. A few of his little charges had been left behind when he had moved a hive. A couple soon found my soft English skin and I received painful stings. Besides the pain, alarmingly I became quite ill and my throat started to swell...I think I was heading for an anaphylactic reaction but we were near a chemist and antihistamines helped. After that I avoided bees and always carried medication with me especially when Ken gave me a lift.

The Hospital Board house which came with the job was adequate. There were two bedrooms, a small lounge, a kitchen and a bathroom. Set at the back of the house and with doors both to a small hall and the house, was my office. Patients could come to see me that way without entering our living area.

At first I had a little concern about driving an ordinary car instead of the van, but I soon became used to it. As I had a new car every couple of years, I had several different makes and became adept at coping with the peculiarities of Toyota, Datsun and Holden makes. The roads were so rough, dents and scratches were commonplace, and it was easier to replace than repair the rural cars. I think the urban nurses had our rejects, after they had been to the panel beaters for treatment.

The main roads in my area were tar-seal, but otherwise they were variations of the typical New Zealand country roads. They were mostly covered with rough shingle, and it was sometimes like driving on a beach. Road repairs generally consisted of a lorry loaded with stones preceding a grader, whose large blade levelled out the piles of shingle manually thrown from the back of the lorry. While touring New Zealand by Bedford van with my family, I had had plenty of practice with these unmade roads but I found a car quite a different vehicle to drive. It was much lighter, even allowing for the nursing equipment I carried. I also was often in a hurry, having a busy day ahead.

Sometimes the camber at the edge was very steep and I soon learned to take corners wide. One day I did not, and the car slid gracefully down the steep gutter between the end of the shingle and the verge. Try as I might I could not get out and had to walk to the nearest farmhouse conveniently within sight. An amused farmer hauled me out by tractor.

Soon after I started my job one morning the car would not start. It was my luck, a patient arrived who knew about cars. We both stuck our heads under the bonnet; 'Ah,' said my saviour, 'it's your ignition solenoid.' There was a detached wire, and he showed me where it should be re-attached by a clip.

I had reason to bless this man again some weeks later.

One of my first visits had been to an outlying farm where a patient needed stitches removed. I had arrived later than planned, as I was yet unused to the time it took to find the addresses given. There were never any road numbers and often no names either on the mailboxes. Instructions were sometimes extremely casual. 'Oh, it's the third farm on the left after the road bends; the roof is painted green.' After several false calls and by asking anyone I saw in the fields, the place was at last located, only to be told, 'ah yes, I forgot we had the roof re-painted red last month.'

In this case I attended to the farmer's wife and went out to my car. No keys. I searched my pockets, work bag and ignition, then went back into the house to see if I had dropped them. Still no keys. My patient's sister who was staying came out to look, too.

'Here they are, in your lock in the boot, Sister!' I felt an idiot. I was sure this would go round the village.

A couple of days later my patient was brought to the surgery for me to check the wound. There was no mention of my previous incompetence and they soon left. Almost immediately there was a knock on my door. 'So sorry to bother you, Sister, but the car won't start; can we use your phone to ring for help?'

'Sure, but may I have a little look first? I know a bit about cars.' I am not sure what prompted my rashness, but I wanted to redeem myself if possible.

I stuck my head under the bonnet, and sure enough there was this wire sticking up like mine had been. I remembered what the man had done and did likewise.

The car started, and I was exonerated.

On another occasion I was not as lucky. My car had just been in to have the rust removed and a paint job done, and I was pleased to have it back. It was a Datsun 180b and I had become quite fond of it as it handled well, though it was not always easy to get all the equipment I needed for patients, in the boot.

My patient was just off the main road which ran through my village and on to a town further north, and quite busy. Her drive was steep and had a deep, wide ditch either side. It was quite difficult, and I had to slow down to bottom gear and do a sharp left turn. I looked in my mirror and saw a big old heavy car close behind. I had been indicating a left turn for some time, but wound my window down and made hand signals as well. In my mirror I saw the other car draw back, so concentrated on the turn. The next thing I knew was a tremendous crash and jolt behind, my head cracked hard back on the headrest and my glasses flew off under the pedals. Almost without thinking I jammed my foot on the clutch to engage neutral, as the car shot through the air landing on the two off-side wheels. I could feel the whole vehicle start to roll and instinctively eased my foot back on the clutch engaging bottom gear. The car rode up the ditch on two wheels, spun up onto the road and landed back on all four wheels again. I disengaged the engine and slammed on the brakes. Shakily I got out of the car and looked back. How we had not rolled, I will never know.

An old man was getting out of his car and hobbled towards me; 'Are you OK? So sorry; so sorry; my foot slipped on the accelerator instead of the brake!'

I took the man's details and got back in the car and found it would still go, despite the back being buckled.

I did not realise how badly I had been affected until that evening. I finished my day's work and reported the accident to my superiors.

The next day I could hardly move; I had severe whiplash that was to affect me for many years to come, but I realised how lucky I had been, and blessed my quick reactions.

4/6

The Auckland Extramural hospital was run on slightly different lines from most district nursing services. Normally the local Health Authorities controlled everything, from the nurses to equipment on loan. The Extramural Hospital was under the direction of the Auckland Hospital Board. They rightly claimed that in many cases the patient could and should be treated at home with no detriment to the standard of care.

Besides supervising the nurses, the Extramural Hospital offered the services of social workers, occupational therapists and bed-linen loans (if there was a continence problem or if a severely ill patient could not cope with the washing; this did not include personal items). Some equipment was also available, such as commodes, crutches, bed cot-sides and even hospital beds.

It was generally the district nurses' job to assess a patient's needs and start refer to the applicable service. We nurses also gave total care in the home, from cutting old folk's toe nails; bathing or showering; injections of all sorts; dressings; training relatives to cope; to care of the dying and laying out the dead. There was always, at least one terminal case on my books, either from cancer, a stroke, or just old age. Then, of course there was not just one patient, but the whole family. I was fortunate in being on my own, I could decide to visit as many times I could manage.

Soon after I began my rural district work, the Auckland Hospital Board introduced a new system of day-release operations for less serious cases, such as varicose veins, removal of cysts and benign lumps, and hernias. This released beds for more severe cases but put a heavier load on the district nurses and families.

Patients were instructed to starve from the night before and had their operations early in the morning. They were then discharged into our tender care by early evening.

This of course meant evening and sometimes night calls if the patient was in pain as they often were, especially the hernia cases. It is at best a painful procedure, and we usually had several calls a night from distraught relatives, as the patient needed painkiller injections. After a few adverse reports from the nurses, hernia patients were eventually kept in for a night or two.

We also worked many weekends and public holidays, including Christmas Day and of course if a patient was on twice a day treatment, evening visits would be necessary. Besides this I often held late afternoon clinics for those who were fit enough to attend, so I was always busy. Sometimes it was almost too much to have to get out of a warm bed to do a night call. I seldom met other traffic at night on the country roads and of course it was pitch black. Once I was nearly dozing off at the wheel and saw a brown shape caught in the headlights. Skidding to a halt, I realised a cow was bedded down and wearily had to climb out of my car and shoo it onto the roadside.

I was wide awake after that.

This was long before mobile phones and although I did have an answerphone in the office, I did not have a remote access. Many were the times I returned from visiting a patient at the further reaches of my district, only to have a message to visit someone in difficulty, or a new patient in the area I had just left.

One of the main disadvantages of 'living on the job,' was during my days off. Quite often when the relief nurse was out on her calls and I was catching up on housework or sitting in the garden, there would be a ring on the surgery doorbell. I was tempted to ignore it, but it could just be an emergency.

'Oh, Sister, my dressing has all come undone.' Or 'Nurse, I'm due for me injection, just thought I'd save time and call in.' So what do you do but change that dressing or give that injection, of course.

There was also clerical work to attend to. Besides personal notes, there was a card index system which kept visits up to date. As soon as a patient had been seen, the card was put into an appropriate slot for next day or week or longer. I found this very useful as I could keep track of patients' families too after a death, just popping the card for a visit in a month or so.

I used to dread the end of the month as I had to tally my visits. Each day I had to fill in forms denoting type of visit; medical, surgical, maternity, paediatric or geriatric. The visits, on a separate sheet also had to be divided into time spent giving treatment, including travelling time; from 15 minutes, 30 minutes, an hour, to over an hour. These all had to tally, which mine rarely did.

Maths had not been my strongest subject at school.

I greatly enjoyed the variety of work and the elasticity of my hours. It did mean Ken and I saw less of each other, which suited us both. Already we were drawing apart, although I did not realise at the time what would lie ahead. We had talked of splitting up for a trial in the future, but with Roy still not in secondary school we agreed to delay any decision. There were too many days when we hardly spoke, but there were no arguments and we just carried on with our lives.

It was an advantage to be working in the community where Roy went to school, though he did not always appreciate it.

Unfortunately for Roy, as I often had his classmates' families as patients, I got first-hand news of goings-on at the local school. I had been surprised my son seldom had homework and I happened to mention it to a girl in his class who had had a small operation. While I took the stitches out, as a distraction I said,

'I'm surprised you don't have homework very often.'

The mother chipped in, 'oh, Judy has lots, don't you dear?'

Judy looked at the stitches I had removed, with relief. 'Oh, yes, but Roy is allowed to stay in at playtime and do his. He says he must do so many chores when he goes home that he doesn't have time in the evening!'

I felt a bit sick, and then angry. 'That's not true, what on earth will people think?' Not generally too worried about public opinion, I did have to have a good public image in this community. I did not want to be seen as a Tartar of a mother. 'Right, I'm off to the school!'

I marched straight to the headmaster's office on arrival, and managed to see his wife who taught the eleven- to thirteen-year-olds in the 'intermediate' section. She was fair but strict, and listened to me without comment, then thoughtfully said,

'I did wonder. He is a bright little boy, but has a rather unusual life, I suppose. He is a bit disruptive in class....'

I could not believe it, my Roy, disruptive? I knew he was forgetful. He seldom gave me the notes about events and parents' meetings until it was too late. I had learned to look in his school bag each evening, just to check.

'Let's go and have a talk with Roy,' she looked at a timesheet, 'they are just finishing a maths class.'

If there had been any doubt, the look on Roy's face as we walked into the class and called him out, told its own story. We all had a little chat, and I controlled my annoyance as best I could. I knew it would do no good to lose my temper. As a Sagittarian, I had a somewhat mercurial temperament. While I did not avidly follow astronomy, I felt there was some merit in 'star signs.' As a 'Libra' Roy is a perfect example of someone trying to balance people and events around him, even to telling fibs, in reality or by omission.

This was one more lesson I had to learn as a mother. Suffice it to say as soon as Roy went up into the intermediate part of his school, in preparation to high school, he never looked back. The headmaster's wife was his teacher and she kept him busy. I think his main problem was boredom as he was such a bright child.

There was another occasion neither of us will forget and made me glad I often popped into the office to check any messages if I was visiting nearby. On this occasion I was concerned to hear the headmaster's anxious voice.

'Sister Davies, I am afraid Roy has had an accident at school. He needs to go to hospital, is there any chance you could call in, now?' I noted that I had just missed the call, so rang back.

'What has happened?'

'He had a fall in the playground and has a badly broken arm.'

'I am on my way.' I quickly phoned my superiors and morning's patients, fortunately none of them urgent and drove quickly to the school.

The poor lad was sitting white as a sheet in the headmaster's office.

'Never mind an ambulance, I'll take him myself.' Gently I guided my brave son into the back of the car and tried to make him comfortable, loosely strapping the poor deformed arm to his chest. I drove as slowly as I could to the local A&E and reported.

And there we sat.

By this time the poor lad was nearly out of it; the arm must have been very painful as the lower part was almost in an 's-bend'.

'Right, this is where Sister Davies throws her weight about a bit.'

It may have been the uniform or my constant nagging, but we were soon seen, and a young doctor took us into a cubicle.

'Goodness young man, what have you been up to? Fighting?' That was not the best comment as he was not a fighter, but Roy surprised me by saying, 'You should have seen the other boy.'

'Yes, well, what we'll do is give a few injections under your arm and round about, and straighten you out a bit; how does that sound?'

Roy went whiter if that was possible as we laid him down on a bed. I stood by his head and talked. I do not remember what I said but tried to keep his mind off what was happening. Looking at his dear little face, I had a surge of maternal love. I could not contemplate splitting this family up while he still needed us both.

4/7

I soon became used to driving around my district for most of the day. I loved the open air and wild countryside, although I found it inadvisable in high summer to have my window open...no adequate car air conditioning in those days. Dust would boil in through and start me sneezing and looking as if I had not washed either myself or my uniform for weeks. When it was really hot, I abandoned all but the basic underwear and my uniform dress, having to suffer a sauna with all the windows closed.

If I was not in too much of a hurry, I would steal a little time to stop and relish the quietly whispering pine trees on the road through the Riverhead State forest, delighting at the quick flash of red and blue of a flock of parakeets. Or if I was visiting in Muriwai Beach, take a brisk walk on the black sand beach, returning to my car to rub the salt spray off my spectacles and comb my tangled hair before visiting my patients.

Coupled with this I derived great pleasure in the challenge this type of work offered me. I found the different patients fascinating as I had always been interested in people. Even the most difficult ones usually had some reason for that attitude, although I had to admit it was not always possible to change their outlook.

Over the seven years I was to hold my position as rural district nurse, a few of my patients became friends. Sometimes the treatment went on for a long time and it was impossible not to become close.

Angela had five children and somewhere along the years she had developed an intestinal abscess. This was so persistent, it never healed. It became a low-grade infection which pushed up a sinus, a sort of safety valve, to the skin surface. It was necessary to keep this sinus open or the pus built up causing trouble. It was my job to do this by probing into the small hole in Angela's abdomen to release any collected pus with a silver probe instrument. By this time pre-sterilised dressing packs had replaced the old system, and instruments were sterilised at a central department in the hospitals, so life was easier.

For a long time, our visits were daily and Angela and I enjoyed our meetings. One day she asked, 'what do you do about lunch, Chris?'

'I usually take sandwiches and stop when I am hungry, why?'

'Well, I was thinking, I am usually on my own. If it fits in come and have lunch with me, and don't forget to bring your swimming togs!'

So, when I was not too rushed, I spent a delightful half hour or so after my patient's treatment having a swim in her pool and a light lunch. There certainly were a few perks to this job.

Sometimes it was difficult to give treatment; not because it was painful, as mercifully the area we had to probe was so scarred most of the nerve-endings were dead.

The problem was Angela's waterbed.

As our relationship developed, so we had a lot of banter and if Angela got a giggling attack while on the waterbed, it was just impossible to insert a thin probe until she had calmed down.

I needed to keep my patient happy as she was, not surprisingly, prone to depression with no apparent end to her problem. She had been in and out of hospitals many times; had innumerable courses of antibiotics and was also on anti-depressants. Her family were all married or away at university and her husband was no help, as he was a jogging addict and keen on 'keeping fit.' I had the impression he thought it all a fuss about nothing.

During one of my patient's spells in hospital I wrote a little rhyme and illustrated it to cheer her. We nurses had been given written instructions outlining a district nurse's responsibilities and I based my offering on those. We were told to be always courteous, and make sure we were welcome; to give injections as painlessly as possible; to be tidy with dressings; to make showers an enjoyable experience and generally be good examples of impeccable behaviour. Angela loved it, but when I put it on the nurses' notice board during an occasional meeting I had to attend, my supervisor was not as pleased with it.

'The district nurse is on the way; shout hooray, shout hooray,
She drives her car so very well, truth to tell, truth to tell.
No doubt a min'string angel she, as all can see, as all can see.
Patients love to see her call; welcome all, welcome all.
To serve the public is her joy; 'tis her employ, her employ.
Injections given with no pain; call again, call again.
Dressings quick and neatly done; oh what fun, oh what fun;
Her showers are a pleasure too, without ado, without ado.
See, here she comes and rings the bell.
So lock the door and run like h......l.'

******

Another family I became fond of was an elderly couple living in a wonderful house high above the famous surfing beach of Muriwai. Each time I called to give Ethel a bath I had to stop and admire the cascading white rollers pounding onto the black sand beach. A mist of spray blew as far as the eye could see, until the sea, sand and sky blended into one mystical area. The gannets nesting nearby circled further out to sea with flashes of white, black wingtips and bright golden heads catching the sun. They would dive like jet propelled arrows into the waves, later emerging with a wriggling fish in their beaks.

Jack had been in the merchant navy and said his house was as good as being at sea. Ethel his wife had what we now call Alzheimer's; then, Senile Dementia. I saw from their photos strewn through the house she had been very beautiful, and Jack was still devoted to her. She was now extremely stubborn and needed all my patience to coax her to sit in the bath. Sometimes it took half an hour, so I also used to time my visit at lunchtime. If we shared a lunch, Ethel saw me as a friend or even one of their children and so was a little more amenable.

One night I had a phone call from Jack. 'It's Ethel, she's not moving. I think…I think she may be dead.'

'Have you called the doctor?'

'No, please can you come first. If she's dead, he can't do anything can he?'

I quickly dressed, told Ken where I was going and grabbed my bag, just checking who her doctor was. Sure enough the poor woman had slipped away in her sleep, so I rang the doctor and waited until he arrived. I attended to the 'Last Offices' as we called the laying out, but I could see Jack was very upset.

'Do you want me to stop a while? Let's have a cup of tea.' I stayed until the dawn light crept magically over the beach, letting the old man reminisce over their life together. I realised Jack had been away for long spells and wondered if that contributed to their continued lifelong love.

As I was leaving…I had to get back to sort my visits for the day, Jack suddenly grabbed my hand. 'You will still drop in for a spot of lunch now and again, won't you?'

Jack left to live with his son in the South Island. Later, on holiday near Nelson where he now lived, I called into see the old man. He was still his spritely, smartly dressed self, but he admitted to me some of the light had gone out of his life. I wondered what it would be like to love someone as deeply.

I was to discover that, one day.

4/8

Not all my patients caused me sadness. Some families gave much entertainment and were an education on how to live contentedly, although from the outside their life seemed totally chaotic. In the end sometimes there was sorrow. By the nature of our work, we nurses were involved with all aspects of the human condition.

Such a family were the Gregsons. The old grandmother, Lily, was my patient but I could not help but be involved with the whole family. The pivot and mainstay was her daughter Rosie. A stocky typical farmer's wife in appearance, with ruddy face and cheerful determination she kept the extended family going.

With the diagnosis of 'Huntington's chorea', a hereditary condition manifested as involuntary and often violent movements of arm and facial muscles, Peter had to give up farming. The whole family moved to a rambling bungalow with outhouses, an extended yard all around, a paddock and a deep stream at the back. There were several pine trees behind the house and Peter was in the process of having them felled, to sell as firewood. The trouble was, he decided to chop the kindling himself. I never quite got used to the sight of an axe waving around in every direction held by this weaving heavily built man. I was expecting him to chop something other than the log in question, but he never did. Somehow the kindling piles grew, un-contaminated by stray pieces of dog, cat, chickens, or himself.

During my visits to bath Lily, I met the rest of the family. There were two grown children. Charlie was the eldest and was away from home most of the time, only appearing to hand his mother wads of money. I never asked what he did. Christina was living away from home too with a partner, and I saw her occasionally, wondering how she had managed to keep her fresh beauty with the chaotic childhood she must have had. I could see the same beauty, now faded, in her mother.

Frank was about sixteen and a devoted mechanic. If it did not work, then there was a chance Frankie could mend it. The trouble was, he was accident-prone and frequently cut or bruised himself and I did but wonder if he had inherited his father's illness. It was often my job to try and change a dressing or remove stitches. but he was seldom at home when I needed to give treatment.

I soon learned there was no point in insisting.

'Where is Frankie, this time Rosie?' I'd wearily ask.

'Oh, down the back in that old banger, I think.'

So, I went to locate my patient, sat him in the back seat of the car and did what needed to be done. Not perhaps the standard procedure, but I had little choice.

The final member of the family was a delightful four-year-old, Poppy.

'Was she an afterthought?' I asked Rosie, one day.

'Oh no, dear, she's Christina's.' She looked round to see the child could not hear, 'she thinks I'm her mum, but I'm really her granny. Christina had a little mishap; I didn't want to spoil her life, so I adopted Poppy.' She touched my arm, 'you won't say anything will you. I'll tell her when she's ready.'

'No, of course not. It's none of my business.' I warmed to this generous person.

The old woman, Lily, was a different story. A cantankerous, quarrelsome, unpleasant person, I never really liked her. For all her daughter did for her, she spent my whole visit complaining about Rosie. I was to give her a bath and change her clothes, but it was an uphill task. I suppose it was not her fault the bathwater was gritty and the clothes she produced as stained as the ones we removed, but whatever I did was wrong.

Mind you the house was like a gigantic jumble sale. Piles of clothes were scattered everywhere. Chickens, cats, and dogs wandered in and out of each room and I was hard put to find something to fit the old lady. Once I brought a sack of clothes from someone who was clearing a relative's home, hoping to improve matters. They disappeared into the piles, never to be seen again.

On one of my visits Poppy ran up holding a kitten for me to see. It was tiny, and I wondered how old it was. Its tiny pink mouth opened in a loud plea, and I tried to show the little girl how to hold it properly.

The following visit I saw Poppy again. 'How's the little kitten, Poppy?'

'Oh, it's sleeping. It keeps sleeping and won't wake up.'

Concerned, I asked to see it. Lying stiff and very dead the tiny mite was wrapped in one of the bundles of clothes.

'Oh dear, Poppy, I am afraid it is dead.' The little girl began to cry.

'Tell you what, let's have a proper funeral.' We found a box; Frankie made a cross and Rosie, Poppy and I marched to a corner of the yard and dug a hole, putting a bunch of wildflowers on the tiny mound.

My visits continued each week although I often wondered what good I was doing. There was covert animosity between old Lily and Peter, but Rosie acted as a buffer. Until one day she was away visiting a friend with Poppy. As I got out of my car, I could hear Peter shouting, swearing and a banging on the door and I saw he had his axe in his hand, threatening to chop the old woman into pieces.

'Now then Peter, what's all this about?' I kept my distance and the car door open but did not think I was in any danger; we had always got on well.

'Silly old bat thinks I want to rape her.' To my relief he threw down the axe. 'She's as mad as a hatter. You are welcome to her.' With that he shambled off and sat on a nearby log.

'Lily, it's me, district nurse; let me in.'

The door opened a crack, and I saw Lily with a huge carving knife in her hand standing on the other side.

'I'll get the randy bugger; see if I don't.'

I realised I could not leave the two together, so quickly packed a few clothes in a plastic bag and left a note for Rosie.

'Let's go for a little ride and see what can be done.' Lily came quietly as I drove to the local small hospital where I knew they had respite beds, and just hoped they would take her in for a few days.

They were able to take the old lady for a few days, and she was assessed. It was decided to offer the family a place in the local nursing home. Here she thrived, making friends with others there and when I called to see her, she was a different person; clean and almost content.

'Mind you I still say he was up to no good,' she declared as I left.

Up to no good or not, Peter came to a sad end a few months later. I had stopped calling regularly but heard from other patients his body had been found in the stream at the bottom of their adjoining paddock.

His condition had been getting worse, and it will never be known how he met his end. The coroner's report said he had had a heart attack but there was also water in his lungs.

Rosie continued to look after her depleted family. I called in to see her occasionally, but some of the life in her had gone. For all the chaos of her earlier life, she had thrived on it.

A little while after, I heard on the local grapevine poor Rosie had been diagnosed with breast cancer. I was so sad for this woman who was such an example of how to make the best of whatever life dealt.

Sorrow was not often far from my day-to-day visits; sometimes arriving when least expected.

Tony and Judy Harris had first been on my books a year previously. I had been asked to visit Judy as a post-natal following the birth of her first child and was surprised to find the father, Tony, at the house also.

'I thought I'd stay at home and give a bit of paternal support,' he explained, 'anyway my foot is hurting a bit, must have trodden on something.' He said he worked at the local Forestry, replanting young pine trees. The ground was rough with debris of the old, felled trees about.

I visited for a week to make sure mother and baby were settling, but noticed Judy was a little distracted, and wondered about post-natal depression. I watched her care for the baby, but there did not seem to be any tension there. Finally, I asked; 'Is everything OK. How is Tony's foot?'

Judy turned a worried face towards me. 'That's just it. I sent him to the Doc. and he said Tony must have a ... what's it called ... a bio-something.'

'Biopsy, do you mean?'

'Yes, his father died of cancer, so they aren't taking any chances. Do you think he'll be OK?'

'Yes, I am sure it is just a formality.'

My words came back to haunt me in the months to follow. It was cancer; a particularly invasive type which spread to the groin rapidly.

The wound in the groin would not heal, and I called for daily dressings over the next few weeks. Judy was coping well, and they were both positive until the fateful day of the discovery of more lumps under his arms and the other groin.

Tests and examinations showed the cancer had advanced. There was no hope.

My visits gradually increased to twice daily. I did all I could, but inevitably it became too much for Judy, with a young child to care for as well. Her mother lived a long way away, her father was dead, and she did not get on with her in-laws, although they visited regularly.

I took Judy on one side after I had made Tony comfortable, and said, 'I really think Tony should go into the hospice for a while, you just aren't sleeping, and the baby needs you too.'

Eventually Judy agreed, but whether it was the move or just that he gave up, Tony died a few days later. I called in to see Judy just to see how she was coping and I was concerned she was too well-controlled.

'Is there no-one you can go to, Judy?'

'I'm alright; I'm alright. Just leave me alone!'

There was not much else I could do except contact the social worker, who promised to keep an eye on her.

A few weeks later, I met the social worker and asked after Judy Harris.

'It's a good job you referred her. She was told to move, as it was a Forestry house and as her husband was no longer an employee, she could not stay. It must have been the last straw.'

I felt sick as I was afraid what was coming next. 'She tried to gas herself and the baby; luckily I had decided to drop in, just in time.'

'Will she be alright?'

'Yes; I think so. The in-laws have taken mother and baby in. Whatever the problem was has been resolved, but oh dear, how sad, how sad.'

4/9

I had become used to dogs during my life. My father had a big Alsatian when I was little, then while I was at school we had a delightful Welsh collie, who was my constant companion. I thought I would have no problems with the farm dogs on my nursing rounds, but they were quite a different story. Bred solely for work with stock, these animals were kept outside chained to their kennels, unless needed. At the times I visited they were working and tended to be loose round the yard and fields. I was often confronted by a slobbering pack of wild-looking animals, milling round the car as I tried to get out. The trick was to show no fear and to swear loudly at them. With memories of my theatre nursing days during my training, I had picked up a few choice words, and it usually worked.

The worst offenders were the little yappy dogs owned by young families I had to check on post-natal visits. One black and white nasty little Jack Russel used to stand on the inside of the gate barking furiously, and not let me in. If I did brave it, the vicious animal made a dive for my heels. After a couple of nips I had enough. The hard wooden case I carried with equipment for my visit had sharp corners and I discovered it was a useful deterrent, especially when his teeth contacted the wooden corner instead of my soft skin. After a couple of those contacts, the dog dived under the house, and I was able to carry on with my work. Every time he saw me after that, he just yelped and disappeared under the house. Problem solved.

The sign 'Beware of the dog' on the gate of a new patient did not therefore cause me too much concern. I was not so sure about another notice nailed to a tree 'Trespassers will be shot on sight.'

I had been asked to visit by one of the GPs. 'Go and have a look at 'Beaky' Smith, will you, Chris. A neighbour is concerned he is not looking after himself. You may need to call in the social workers but let me know what you think.' This was typical of many referrals and worked well in our community. Sometimes the patient went onto our weekly shower list; sometimes there was more of a problem which needing experienced intervention.

In this case I climbed the five-bar gate and started to walk over the grassy paddock towards a small shack set by a stream. It was a glorious day, bright and sunny with spring-like weather. There was a hill behind with a scattering of native trees; the star shape of punga and upright thrust of cabbage trees surrounded by the fuzzy bushes of tee-tree, now frosted with the white of blossom. For all that I revelled in the weather I was keeping a sharp ear and eye out for the dog and a possible shotgun.

There was no sound as I approached the cottage, but the door was ajar. I knocked hard, holding my nursing bag handy as protection just in case. Pushing at the door I called out, 'Mr Smith, hello; district nurse.' I was a little concerned, but reasoned that if the man was ill, the dog would still be around. I ventured into the room which was surprisingly tidy, with a fire laid in the hearth and a table and chairs in the middle of the room. Old, but clean lino was on the floor, and I could see a bed made up in an adjoining room. Suddenly I heard a barking behind me a little way away and retreated outside, shading my eyes to look up the hill. I could just see them against the glare of the sun; the tall, big-nosed man with a long shepherd's crook in his hand and a tattered coat flapping round him and the dog running fast towards me. I stood my ground.

After all I had a good reason to be there.

The dog reached me first, and stopped barking to move towards me, sniffing. I stood quite still and spoke soothingly to him. 'My you're a nice fellow. I am sure you don't want to bite me, do you?' I think he could smell my dog Bitsa on me as the sheepdog started slowly to wag his tail.

'So, young lady, what can I do for you?' It was not what I had expected, and neither was the man standing before me. While in his early seventies, he still looked wiry and lean; face tanned to a leathery brown and thick curling white hair blown by the wind.

'Er, the doctor asked me to pop in on my way past to see if you needed any help. He said you'd had a touch of bronchitis.'

'No, I'm OK. I bet it was that nosy neighbour Betty Thomson sent you round.' He gave a cough, 'people should mind their own business.' He walked past me and pushed the door open. 'Well, you've been inside already, you might as well have a cup of tea. We were just going to have one, weren't we, old Bob.' I could feel the dog's wet nose sliding up and down my leg, so decided to accept the offer and moved into the cottage again.

While he made the tea, Beaky Smith told me a few stories of the old days when he had been a sheep musterer; now he only had a few head up on the hill but attended them as in the old days.

'It was the early lambing ye see, had to stay out with them, got a bit of a chill.' He took a small bottle from a shelf behind him and slopped a little in his tea, offering it to me; I shook my head. 'No thanks, not while I'm working.' I took a sip of the strong brew, 'which brings me to my visit.' I was not sure how to broach the subject. 'We, that is the doctor, wondered if you needed any help with showering and things.'

'Now that's an offer it's hard to resist; wish I was a bit younger.' I caught the twinkle in his faded blue eyes and felt myself blushing. 'Anyway, I don't have a shower,' he took a swig at his fortified tea. 'If I need a wash, I pop up to the hot pools up in Parakai; soon cleans me up.'

I thought of the times our family had gone up to swim in the hot thermal pools, and inwardly shuddered. I looked up in time to see the smile in Beaky's eyes and was not sure if I was having my leg pulled.

'Got ye there, didn't I,' he chuckled. 'Not sure if I was having ye on?' I found the man strangely charismatic and wondered how he had ended up on his own in this tiny shack with just a few sheep and a dog. I had enjoyed my visit and asked if it would be alright for me to pop in now and then.

'Yes, Sister, if ye like, and if any of your posh patients have a spare coat, I could do with one.'

I had been thinking of a pile of clothes recently left at my office. I was sure there was a winter coat among them and had wondered how I could offer it to Beaky Smith without offence. Obviously, I need not have worried.

Beaky Smith's obvious enjoyment of the idea of a nurse giving him a shower was not a new one to me. Sometimes our male patients thought our services included more than attending to medical needs. Occasionally when helping with a shower, the interest of a male patient was obvious, and I realised how vulnerable we nurses were. In these cases, I had no hesitation in arranging for a male nurse to visit from headquarters.

On one occasion I did not see the writing on the wall and became a little too involved with a charming orchard-owner.

I met Mario Ponti after he had a hernia operation when his wound needed attention. He and his wife Helen were about my age, and it was a change to have a patient who was not terminally ill or old. I was pleased when they became friends and even Ken, who was not particularly sociable, joined in. We had the occasional barbecue together and if Mario flirted with me a little, I thought it was all part of the fun; he was a very attractive Italian and I had to admit I was flattered by his attention.

This went on for a year or two, but I was becoming a little uneasy with the obvious attentions of this highly sexed man. What began as a light-hearted game gradually came to a head after he had a second operation to remove a cyst on his leg. I was less than comfortable giving treatment and tried to make sure his wife was around when I changed the dressing.

One day as I arrived, I could see she was in the orchard picking fruit some distance away.

'Ha, so at last I have you to myself!' Mario exclaimed, I hoped in jest as I arrived and parked the car.

'I'll just let Helen know I am here,' I said as I put my bag down in the bedroom where I usually changed the dressing.

'Not yet, we don't need her just at the moment do we, Christabelle.' I had learned to dislike his nickname for me.

Before I knew what he was up to Mario shut the bedroom door and wrapped his arms round me, trying to kiss me on the mouth. 'Stop it Mario, don't be silly!'

'Come on, you've been dying for it; now's our chance. Helen will be out there for another hour.' I started to panic, realising perhaps I had been a little too friendly with a man I hardly knew.

'No, I'm sorry, Mario. You've got the wrong idea.' Then I heard the crunching of gravel on the drive outside as a vehicle drew up next to mine.

'Hi, Chris, are you there?' It was Ken's voice, and for once I was delighted to hear it.

I pushed Mario onto the chair. 'I'll be back to do the dressing in a minute' I said as I bolted through the door, leaving it open.

'I thought you might be here. A message came in, so I thought I'd try and find you.' He stepped into the room and handed me a slip of paper. Ignoring my flushed face he said 'Hi' to Mario and got back into the van.

I quickly did the dressing, leaving the door propped wide open and telling Mario there was no need for me to call again.

4/10

Living and working in the same community meant we were well known, but it was not so different from our time in Sark, as sometimes my professional life overlapped into my private one.

While it was not the accepted practice to talk to a doctor about illnesses past and present in a public situation, no such reserve apparently applied towards a nurse.

'Ah, Chris, let me show you how well my wound has healed.' Or, 'Sister I just wonder if you could give me some advice about ...' became common approaches. I was really my own worst enemy, as I was usually interested, but Ken became very tired of the constant interruptions in the few social occasions we attended together.

One community activity we both enjoyed was with the Scouting movement. We early enrolled Roy in the local pack, and it gave him the opportunity to meet others of his own age. Ken was very keen, as he had been with his youth club in London, and soon became involved. His patience and understanding was much appreciated. He spent considerable time encouraging the boys to work for their 'badges.' For these they had to have certain instruction on a topic, say cooking, and then take a test. If passed, a special badge was awarded in a small ceremony and then sewn onto their uniform.

One day Ken asked if I could help with the first-aid badge.

'Er, well, what will I have to do?' I asked, in a little trepidation. I had just completed a Red Cross course but facing about 30 little boys was a little daunting.

'Just tell them the basics and then you must ask each one some questions. Simple!'

Ken may have thought it simple, but I was not good with children unless they were ill, but I did not want to let the Scouts down. On the allotted day, and with more preparation than I had done for some of my exams, I confronted three rows of little boys sitting cross-legged on the floor of the Scouts' Den. I had rigged up an 'accident' using red paint and *cello tape*, but kept it hidden to begin with. At first I needed to start with the basics.

'Now, supposing you come across an accident, what is the first thing you should do?' Hands reached up. From 'call a policeman,' to 'run for help', we established it was important to make sure neither they nor their patient could come to further harm. I told them of an occasion I had heard of, when someone ran off for help, leaving a person to choke on blood from a bitten tongue. I talked on some more with basic instructions on how to cope with every-day problems. 'Remember you are just first aiders, not medics; all you have to do is to stop things getting worse before someone comes to help.'

Suddenly whipping my hand from behind me, I produced a realistic-looking gash on my hand, with what looked like a piece of wood sticking out of it. There were gasps and several 'yuks'! 'Look what has just happened; I need help!' I pretended to feel faint and was delighted at the response. No-one tried to remove the piece of wood and they were all helpful until they realised I was putting it on. There was much relieved laughter. I had surprised myself by having a stimulating evening. They were a great bunch of boys and of course I passed them all for their badges. It became an annual job for me, which I enjoyed over the years.

It was not very long before my first aid was called upon in a real situation.

Barbara Stewart lived in a small flat in her son Tony's large sprawling bungalow just outside my village. She recently had a hip replacement, but something had gone wrong and an abscess had developed on the suture-line. I was asked to call in and assess the situation, and dress the wound as needed.

We immediately developed a rapport, and I loved this white-haired old lady's independence and wicked sense of humour. For some time I called in daily to attend to the dressing, and Tony got into the habit of popping in to see how the wound was progressing as he was very close to his mother. From the first we made friends, and I found his drawling Kiwi accent and sparkling bright blue eyes attractive. I had seen him a few times at the indoor bowling club I joined soon after I arrived, but not really got to know him. After a while, as the wound was still pouring out offensive pus despite Barbara's being on antibiotics, I decided to take a swab.

'We'll send this off to the lab and get a report to your doctor. Maybe you need a change of antibiotics.'

Sure enough, it was found she had become resistant to the antibiotics and a new, potent one was prescribed.

'It will have to be by injection: stay with Mrs Stewart for a while, sometimes people have had a slight reaction to this antibiotic. It is a new one but maybe we can get rid of the infection for good and all,' the doctor instructed me. This instruction undoubtedly saved Barbara Stewart's life.

I apologised for the first painful injection and suggested we have a cup of tea as Tony had arrived for his daily visit. Barbara insisted on going into her tiny kitchen to make the tea, as I put my equipment away.

Suddenly there was a crash and Tony dashed into the kitchen.

'Oh my God, quick Chris, it's Mother, she's collapsed; I don't think she is breathing!'

I only needed a moment to realise my patient had an anaphylactic shock reaction to the antibiotic. I felt for a pulse at the neck.

Nothing.

'Phone for an ambulance, quick Tony,' I exclaimed as I laid Barbara on her back and loosened her clothing, tipping her head back and whipping out her false teeth so that I could begin artificial respiration. I searched again for a pulse and feeling none, I gave her chest two sharp bangs, and continued with resuscitation. I had done this before, as well as having first aid instruction. After what seemed like forever, I felt a faint flutter under my fingers, which grew gradually stronger. As soon as I was sure Barbara was back with us, I rolled her on her side into the recovery position and covered her with a blanket Tony had brought me.

'The ambulance is on the way: God, that was a close call.' He was white and shaking. I had to admit I was a little shaken, too. It had happened so quickly.

In no time at all we heard the sirens approaching and I thanked Heaven that there was an ambulance station in the next village. Soon Mrs Stewart was on the way to hospital accompanied by her son, and I phoned her doctor to report.

'I hope you don't ask me to use that antibiotic again, it seems pretty lethal,' I exclaimed as I was still a little shaken.

'Yes, that is why I advised you to hang around for that reason.'

'Do you mean you suspected that reaction?'

'It was a possibility.' I bit my tongue so as not to say anything I might regret. This doctor was not one I liked working within my area. Of the four I had to deal with, my favourites were a husband-and-wife team who were very supportive and we worked well together. Another was rather casual, and I suspected would not back me on some of the decisions I had to make, and this one who was often down-right rude. He obviously thought nurses were a necessary nuisance to be endured. He came from another country, and it appeared their view of a woman's place in society was low on the social scale. I had several battles in the past with this man, particularly when he was on call at weekends. Often there was only one doctor on duty during weekends and public holidays in my whole area. If I had a terminal patient who was on the verge of needing more painkiller injections, I sometimes needed the dose to be increased. Normally a doctor would call and see the patient, giving a written instruction to the nurse. When there was only one doctor on call in this extended area, it was the practice to give verbal instruction, to be 'written up' later. I was never happy to accept those instructions from this practitioner, as I was not sure he would support me. I usually notified my superiors to make sure I was covered. These were the days before universal litigation, but the medical profession has always been fair game.

Barbara Stewart recovered fully, and the lethal injection did get rid of the persistent infection.

4/11

The terrain of my area was varied; from wild coastal seas to rolling sheep farms; from tidy orchards to increasing numbers of vineyards and from commercial forests to dusty roads with native bush cascading onto the verges. The patients were also diverse, and I never knew what I would find when investigating a referral.

I enjoyed particularly visiting the new mums and babies. They were a light relief from the sometimes-harrowing circumstances of terminal care. Even in this group there was variety. Some homes were well equipped with every modern convenience, while others barely had enough to give a safe home for a growing family. Over the seven years of my employment, I visited several new babies in the same families, and I was delighted to see their progress. I enjoyed the couples who were building their own home, often in the deep bush, although it was sometime difficult to find the house, there being nothing as modern as a mailbox or road number. I admired these couples, many of whom favoured the 'alternative lifestyle.' Sometimes I felt sorry for the young mother trying to cope with basic sanitation and a shell of a house without internal partitions, doors or much furniture.

Another place I loved to visit was a Hari Krishna Farm which was established in my area. They farmed with oxen and grew everything organically long before it was the fashion to do so. They were all strictly vegetarian and had a very relaxed attitude to life; mostly adopting Indian dress and spending many hours in prayer and chanting.

I soon learned if I wished to see a patient, I had to give my time of expected visit at least an hour before I planned to call; they had no sense of time. On the other hand, I envied their attitude and found it difficult to return to the hustle of my daily rounds after I had been there. On a few occasions Ken, Roy and I accepted an invitation to one of their frequent festival meals in which they were always giving thanks for something or other.

By the nature of their life the inhabitants of the farm were not well off and were grateful for any donations of food. One autumn there had been a local glut of pumpkins and the farm was given many, which brought about an amusing situation, although it could have had more severe repercussions.

The local social worker had been visiting the farm as well on a routine check and phoned my office one morning as I was about to leave.

'Chris, would you have time to call in to the Hari Krishna Farm today? I am a bit worried about one of the young children there. I think he looks a bit jaundiced.'

'Yes, OK, I am down that way a bit later. Which child is it?'

She named a child I had visited just after his birth a year ago. He had seemed fit and well when I saw him a few weeks previously, but I did as asked. Sure enough when I looked at the little lad his skin was very yellow, although the whites of his eyes were clear.

'Has little Jack been sick, very sleepy or off his food?' I asked the mother, who was sitting in a dark blue plain sari with her son on her knee.

'Oh no, he has been eating very well. Just loves all those pumpkins. He has them mashed up every meal; can't get enough.'

The light began to dawn; 'Er, how long has he been eating them?'

The mother thought for a moment; 'well at least a week I should say, maybe more.'

The poor child had a carotenemia I guessed, which was an overload of carotene in his little system.

'I think Jack has had a bit too much pumpkin, he can't get rid of all that pigmentation.'

'Oh dear is it dangerous?'

'Not yet, but if he continued it could affect the brain tissue. I think it would be best if you stopped giving Jack pumpkin.' I made a note to have a word with one of the doctors, just to check.

I sometimes felt this simplistic outlook to life had some disadvantages. I later had to treat a little boy with bad burns to both hands when he had inadvertently put them under very hot water as he visited a friend's house in a neighbouring farm. At the Hari Krishna Farm they had only cold water in the taps.

Both on the farm and among the 'alternative life-stylers' I had noticed their use of natural medicines and homeopathy. I had always been interested in a more natural approach to treating some illnesses and the recent trauma of Mrs Stewart's toxic reaction to an antibiotic made me read more about it. There was an herbalist and homeopath near where I lived, and I decided to attend classes. It was a complete eye-opener.

I soon learned about calendula (marigold) cream and lotion as a healing agent, arnica cream for bruises and sprains and Bach flower *'Rescue Remedy'* drops and cream, a universal helping hand for all sorts of problems. I was never without these, though of course I had to be careful with their use on patients. Nurses could not prescribe and so I used to give details of their use and the patients had to decide if they wanted to try them.

The concept that the body could be stimulated to heal itself was not new to me. I firmly believed an attitude of mind was paramount in the healing process. In homeopathy I found this was taken a step further. It was believed remedies, chosen correctly for the individual, could stimulate the body to heal itself.

At this time New Zealand was advanced in using complementary medicine and some radical ideas were accepted for us nurses to use. Using natural yogurt and manuka honey for wound and leg ulcer dressings was suggested, and I had the chance to try this on a long-term patient, with some success.

Mrs Roberts was only 55 years but looked older. Her hair was iron-grey, and her sallow face lined from constant pain. Dark shadows under her eyes told of sleepless nights and she had to use a walking frame around the house. Her daughter Maisie at 30 could almost have been her sister. Her long plaid skirts reached to her ankles, while her shapeless upper body was encased in plain blouses and sloppy sweaters. Her mousy hair was permed to a frizz, and I never saw her wear makeup on her pale thin face in the time that I attended her mother. This young woman had already succumbed to her mother's affliction of arthritis. She had to use an elbow crutch when she left the house, which she rarely did.

It was not until I knew Mrs Roberts well she told me the whole sad story of her youngest daughter.

'It was five years ago, I'll never forget it,' she told me one day while I was attending to her daily dressing. 'I'd sent Maisie into the city centre with the car to do some last-minute shopping for Christmas. It was the first one since her dad died; thought it might take her mind off it,' Ethel gestured me to a chair as I had finished her treatment.

'It was a Saturday afternoon for goodness's sake, you'd think a young girl would be safe!' A cup of tea was put in front of me and she sat opposite me at the table, 'it happened in the multi-story car park. There were a couple of them, bailed her up in a corner and ... I can't say it ... raped her!' I reached over and touched her hand, but she pulled away.

'I am so sorry...' I began.

'They never found out who it was. No-one went to her help. Can you imagine that?'

'I can understand why she is so shy and retiring. It must be hard to get over something so terrible ... but,' I said.

As if the floods were opened Ethel Roberts continued, 'that's not the worst of it. Nine months later little Bobby was born. He was a lovely baby from the beginning, but Maisie wouldn't even look at him,' she took a drink of her tea, now gone cold, and pushed it away. 'I couldn't let my first grandchild go to strangers, whoever his father was.' She got up and poured another cup of tea for herself. I said nothing. 'My older daughter Penny and her husband adopted him. So I see him often; she has two others now too, but they think Bobby is their brother.'

I did not know what to say, but Mrs Roberts had not finished. 'Then the poor girl started to get this blessed arthritis soon after the birth. The doctors say it is the shock. I just hope she does better than me.'

Mrs Roberts was another patient with complications from an infected hip replacement operation. It was about this time there had been publicity about the use of natural yogurt as a healing and anti-pyretic agent. It was suggested the 'good' bacteria in the yogurt would defeat the toxic infection. My patient's forward-looking doctor, instructed me to try this treatment, so I visited daily armed with live yogurt, sterile saline, and a thin catheter. For weeks we syringed the wound and it certainly did seem to reduce the offensive discharge.

Another *'avant guard'* treatment had recently received much publicity and both patient and doctor decided to try its effectiveness too. It had been discovered honey taken from the New Zealand's native Tea-Tree or manuka flowers had a very healing property. We alternated irrigating the wound with diluted manuka honey.

This was long before this wonderful substance became so popular and expensive.

4/12

With this advanced treatment and my increasing interest in 'Complementary medicine' in mind I was pleased when I was approached by my nursing Headquarters about taking a course in community care at the Auckland Technical Collage. This was being offered to all those working in the health field. Just a few nurses were selected, and I was delighted to be one of them. It took a whole academic year on a day-release, each Friday. At the end participants had to present a community profile and give an hour's presentation to the rest of the 40-strong class. A class consisting of doctors, nurses, social workers, and other medical practitioners.

It was quite a challenge and was like the first day at school again. I presented myself on the appointed day at the meeting hall for our introductory talk, eying my fellow-students. They were all shapes and sizes, but mostly about my age I guessed.

There was a slim middle-aged woman standing at one end of the room, dressed in a neat dark suit. 'Now I want you to divide into small groups of eight and sit on the floor in a circle together.' More and more like school days. I could see others were thinking the same by the grins we exchanged.

'OK, now turn to the person next to you,' the slim woman said. 'You have five minutes each to introduce yourselves to each other. No writing anything down. Then in turn you will stand up and tell the rest of us what your partner has said.' Not so easy, and quite a clever way of discovering how well we listened to each other. I realised I was going to learn much in the following few weeks. The next exercise emphasised that.

'Now we all know each other,' our instructress continued, 'let's see how well you know yourselves.' She held up some pieces of paper and pencils. 'I want you to write ten things you *LIKE* about yourselves.'

Judging by the chewed pencil-ends and frowns, others were having the same trouble I was. Now if it was things I did not like about myself, I would have had no problem. 'So, was that hard?' The woman smiled. 'Well, if you don't like yourself, how can you expect others to?'

That has stuck with me for the rest of my life. We are trained from an early age to be self-depreciatory, but I learned that can go too far.

It was a well-constructed course, and we were introduced to many community activities. We had trips out to a Māori Marae and to a Samoan Islanders meeting hall. We sat in on consultations with doctors and health visitors and went on visits with Plunket and Karitane nurses in their care of mothers and babies.

I had met and worked alongside these highly trained nurses in my practice, and it was interesting to learn more about their professions. Working with children from babies through to school age, they assisted parents by supporting and educating at every stage of early childhood development. They held clinics, parenting education classes, drop-in centres, and gave post-natal home visits, usually taking over when we had discharged the baby a week or so after birth.

I had never really differentiated between the Plunket and Karitane nurses when I had dealings with them on my district, but I soon learned they did have different, though sometimes blending functions. While the Plunket nurses had a wider interest and were more general in their care, Karitane trained nurses specifically helped mothers in their home environment; often staying in the home with a new mother if there were problems.

Other class-room instruction was centred round counselling skills. We were paired off, and were instructed in the art of extracting information by observation and the occasional question. By role-playing, we learned never to ask a leading question.

'And remember,' our class tutor told us, 'never ever give advice. It could come back to haunt you.' He explained further, 'listen to what is being said to you, remember your first day? That was a calculated exercise. You can feed back to your client what they have just said to you.' He called out one of the class and gave a 'mock' interview. He skilfully repeated back what had been said, with a prefix 'so what you are saying is. ...' and then followed it with '... and so what do you think you can do about this problem?' In the end the 'client' produced her own solution. It is a technique I have found always works and was invaluable when I held my own 'Healthy Life Clinics,' many years later.

Throughout the course we had all been working on our projects. Studying my community for the profile was fascinating. Originally there had been a Māori settlement and the waterways had been used extensively for movement from one place to another. Then the Chinese had arrived, valuing the rich soil, and establishing orchards and market gardens, growing apples, pears, stone fruit and many vegetables. A little later the Dalmatians or Yugoslavs and Italians had arrived planting vineyards and the first wines were produced. World-renowned names began here as well as many small but select ones.

Light industry moved into the district and acres of pines were planted to feed the growing need for the housing boom. Gradually more industries were spreading from Auckland, and I rightly predicted that in the not-too-distant future the several small villages would be swallowed by the encroaching city.

Our other project to be presented at the end of the course was to give a lecture on a chosen subject. I chose 'alternative cancer treatment.' Not necessarily to advocate it, but to show what was currently available. With my growing interest in complementary medicine, I had been investigating several popular 'alternative' treatments which were in the news. Some were obviously a big 'con' but others appeared to have some merit, if only because they gave terminal patients some control of their lifestyle.

One such was the use of a substance called 'Laetrile'. Extracted from the kernel of a type of apricot, and rich in vitamin B17 it contained natural cyanide. Discussions were raging in the United States of America as to its legal usage. There had been a clinic set up in Mexico and patients flocked there to receive treatment and instruction. New Zealand at that time allowed apricot kernels to be imported for use in cancer treatment, but the Health Department maintained the cyanide was 'dangerous to health'. I could but wonder what further health hazards a patient with terminal cancer could expect.

The administration of Laetrile was only a part of the treatment. Diet, supplements, and emotional outlook all played a part in this 'metabolic therapy'. I scoured the magazines and papers to save articles and discovered several centres where information was available. I read about one woman who had been given six to eight weeks to live, but she had heard about the Mexico clinic and Laetrile and had gone over as a patient. She combined the Laetrile treatment with conventional treatment. Two years later she and her husband founded a Whole Health Centre to help other sufferers. I also contacted a doctor in Auckland who helped her patients with treatment.

For weeks I spent much of my spare time in visiting people and collecting books and publications. It was certainly fascinating, and I wondered why such treatment was not more widely used. When I studied the necessary diet I began to realise it required a lot of energy and determination to follow the regime. Not only did the participant need to have injections of the Laetrile substance and eat a large quantity of apricot kernels but the diet had to be 80 to 90% raw and fresh vegetables.

I obtained a diet sheet. Cooked food could be included but it was all to be strictly vegetarian. The whole aim was to encourage the immune system to strengthen. With this in mind, certain drinks were advocated. *Rejuvelac* was regarded as a useful source of enzymes and was made from fermented wheat. Two cups of wheat were soaked in four cups of water for 24 hours, strained and then drunk throughout the day. This was repeated for up to six days, keeping it in the fridge. I tried it for a few days, but it tasted like an increasingly pungent alcohol-free beer. The diet sheet said fruit juices could be added, but I found that worse.

Another drink was even less palatable, made from wheatgrass. Trays of wheat were grown, after soaking overnight. Allowed to reach to a height of six to eight inches the young shoots were harvested, then put through a juicer and the resulting dark green liquid drunk. I tried this also with even less enjoyment.

Some of the recipes were quite pleasant so I tried them on Roy and Ken. Muesli mixes soaked in fruit juice over night with sultanas and grated apple added were tasty. I enjoyed the nut loaf, though I think the menfolk were not impressed. Cooked food allowed, included a good biscuit recipe and one of a carrot loaf which became a firm favourite for our family.

One thought occurred often to me while studying this treatment. Most of the people who had tried it had been given a poor prognosis. At least with a diet and treatment requiring long preparation and intense personal involvement patients had to take on some responsibility for their personal survival. I also guessed it was those already with a positive attitude who tried it, and I already knew that was a necessary ingredient in recovery from any illness.

For my teaching project I prepared some of the recipes, including wheatgrass juice, a tray of grown wheat and a jar of fermented *rejuvilac*. I was a little nervous standing in front of my mature audience. They were a far cry from 30 little boy scouts, but I had studied my subject well, and prepared some overhead projections and once I warmed to my subject, I quite enjoyed myself. Judging by my reception I had chosen something of interest and the discussion afterwards was stimulating, though I did not have many takers for the *rejuvilac* and wheatgrass juice.

4/13

This treatment would not have been any help for Tania Hughes by the time she was referred for me to visit. The details were blunt and to the point. *'This 40 year old Māori lady has secondary lesions of carcinoma in her lower spine after the primary cancer was removed from the left breast two years ago. All treatment possible has not stopped the inevitable regression. Her doctor has asked for the Extramural Hospital to help in home terminal care.'*

This was followed by vague directions on locating the orchard run by her Scottish husband. I knew the place as it had my favourite road-side fruit and vegetable stall. One of the things I liked so much about my area was the abundance of fresh fruit and vegetables. Piles of apples, pears, peaches, nectarines, kiwifruit, and strawberries in season, as well as all the vegetables I knew, plus more exotic pumpkin and kumara were there for the choosing. An honesty box was usually on the side of the stall, and I never heard of it being stolen.

Occasionally I had met John Hughes and he had a dour, uncommunicative nature so I was a little concerned about how he would accept my help. I drove through the orchard, marvelling at the acres of trees with glistening ripe fruit hanging like so many Christmas baubles. Normally I would have delighted in the clear fresh air blowing rich growing smells through my open car window, but I was a little worried. In a case like this it was essential to gain the trust and co-operation of the relatives of a terminal patient.

My worst fears were realised as I parked in front of the lovely old colonial house set among the trees. The thickset figure I recognised as John Hughes came out onto the front veranda with arms akimbo. I could see he was very annoyed but underneath I suspected this hid a deep distress and anxiety.

'Where have you been nurse? I have been waiting since eight this morning. They said you would call first thing.'

I refrained from the retort I was tempted to make, mentioning the needs of my other patients, but just smiled and said, 'well I am here now, maybe we could go and see your wife if you would like to lead the way?' I thought an apology would put me in the wrong; I decided I would have to stand up for myself with this man.

'She's in here nurse; you look very young, I hope you know what you are doing.' he said, leading the way into the cool interior of the delightful house.

'Actually, it is "Sister".'

'What?'

'I said, I am a highly trained and experienced Queens Institute of District Nursing Sister, Mr Hughes and I will do everything humanly possible to make your wife comfortable,' I looked him in the eye, 'with your help.' I wondered if I had gone too far, as John Hughes went red in the face, then I saw a small tear slide down his weathered cheek. He suddenly sat down on one of the comfortable chairs in the room we had entered.

'I just don't know what to do to make my dear Tania comfortable. It's that awful hole in her back. No-one should have to suffer like that. She was so beautiful.' He coughed and blew his nose. 'This way, n..., I mean Sister,' he looked at me and I saw a little twitch at the corner of his mouth.

As I entered the bedroom my acute sense of smell picked up a sickly-sweet aroma which caused me to shudder: gangrene.

I could see she had indeed been beautiful. The taught skin now stretched over too-prominent cheek bones still had that golden olive glow common to most Māori women. Her hair, still dark and curling, framed her sweet face and the large deep brown eyes gazed out at me with all the mystery of her race. Her smile was delightful and dimpled her cheeks, as the warmth reached her eyes.

'Hello nurse, so good of you to find time to call. Dear John does his best, but you know men!'

'I am sure your husband will make a good nurse once we sort a few things out.' I gave him a wink, which he received with a rueful smile. 'However, if you wouldn't mind your wife ... may I call you Tania ... and I need to have a little chat.' We were left to it, and I wasted no time in discovering of the source of the unpleasant smell.

'Tania, I need to have a look at what is going on down below; I fear there may be a little problem there.'

'Yes, I know; I can't help the smell,' her eyes brimmed with tears. 'I try to keep cheerful for John, but it is hard sometimes.'

I took my patient's hand noting the strong pulse at her wrist. I guessed this would be a long haul as the heart was obviously still working well. 'You are doing just great. There is a lot we can do to make things easier for you both.'

I noticed my patient was in a low double bed. One of the disadvantages of nursing people in their own homes was the lack of an adjustable 'hospital bed.' In some cases it was possible to borrow a bed from the Hospital loan service, which had a back rest and a variable height, and made things more comfortable for both nurse and patient. In this case it looked as if husband and wife were still sleeping in the same bed so I would have to approach this one carefully. In the meantime, I helped Tania roll over.

'It's alright, nurse, I can't feel anything below my waist. They say there is something on my spine cutting off the nerves.' She said this in such a matter-of-fact way that it caught my breath. I was already full of admiration for this brave woman and had to remind myself not to become too involved.

Sure enough, as soon as the lower back and buttocks were exposed, I saw what all nurses dread; a gangrenous bed-sore. The spinal growth was reducing the blood-flow as well as cutting off the nervous system. I cleaned and dressed the area with hydrogen peroxide but realised there was little hope of healing the sore. After giving a blanket bath and change of bedding, I managed to move my patient onto a chair for a short while.

'Chris,' (we had agreed on Christian names), 'pass me my makeup box from my bedside table, would you please?'

Suddenly Tania Hughes gave a short laugh. 'Just look at me, here am I worrying about my makeup, when we know I am dying.' There was no self-pity, just a statement of fact.

Over the weeks Tania took to end her appointment on this earth, I learned to respect and admire this brave lady. She never complained; never became irritable and showed her love for her husband throughout. He in turn became an excellent carer, even learning to give painkiller injections when necessary. I managed to reduce the offensive gangrenous odour by irrigations of peroxide and packing the eventual large cavity with calendula-soaked dressings. The marigold infusion cleaned the area, and if the rest of the body had been functioning properly, I believe the sore would eventually have healed.

In the event the sweet lady left this earth peacefully one night in late autumn. There was to be a Māori Tangi or funeral and I was invited.

Never again: my resolve not to become involved broke and I could not stop the flow of tears as the voices wailed and speeches were made.

It was about this time I became less content with living in the Hospital Board house. My workload was increasing too as the city started to encroach on the areas where we lived. I was finding working full-time exhausting, trying to combine it with being a housewife and mother. Ken did a fair whack and was a good cook. At the age of twelve Roy was also developing an interest in cooking, which I heartily encouraged. Although I was theoretically working five on and two off days, it did not always work out that way. Sometimes it ran to seven days each of twelve hours or more. As so often happens events took the decision out of my hands. I was requested to call and see the District Supervisor 'when convenient.'

'Christine, as you know we have been asked to cut down on expenses,' my superior looked down at the papers and shuffled them, 'and I am afraid one of the items to go is resident accommodation for district nurses. I am sorry but I have been asked to request you to vacate the Hospital Board house as soon as you can make other arrangements.'

I realised it was decision time. Ken and I had discussed my reducing my working hours.

'Actually, Sister, I was going to have a word about cutting my workdays from five to four a week. I have spoken to Hilary and she would be pleased to do an extra day, er, if that would be agreeable?'

My supervisor looked over her glasses at me. 'Well, that would solve the problem in some ways. You would not have been able to stay in the house as a part-timer.' I opened my mouth to dispute the term for the hours I worked but thought better of it.

So it was that we started to look for a house of our own.

4/14

'It will have to be near enough for us both to get to work, and Roy will soon be going to High School, so we will need to be on a school bus route,' Ken remarked thoughtfully as we looked at the Real Estate lists in the local paper. Gradually we whittled it down to a less expensive area in Waitakere, an area on the boundary of my district. We finally settled on a standard single story New Zealand house. It only had one bedroom and a small office, which kept the price low.

'We'll build an extra bedroom over the sloping garden and then we'll have a carport and workshop for me,' Ken decided. This made an ordinary house more attractive. We had the builder erect a small deck and ranch-slider from the new bedroom, and I spent some time on converting the boring garden with flowering shrubs and fruit trees. We spent our spare time redecorating, and even Roy had a go at wall-papering his own room.

With all I had in my life I should have been content, but I was sometimes restless. I was concerned for the health of my father in England whose Parkinson's disease was getting worse and I wrote to my parents often.

The less hours and our move to a new house reduced the tension which had gradually been building in my daily life. It was great to be able to return home and switch off. I was still on call and had to divert messages to my private phone number, but I was out of the office and not tempted, as I had been before, to pop in and sort a problem which could wait until the next day.

I had hoped I would be happier to spend more time with my husband, but we still grew apart and even agreed to have separate beds in our large new bedroom. Ken had always been a heavy snorer and as the years passed it became worse and irritated me more and more. I knew he could not help it, because of his asthma and polyps in his nose but I was tired of having to block my ears each night. I wondered how much longer we could go on.

Roy was growing up and had started secondary school. As predicted, he was a bright lad, showing an interest in computers and saving up to buy his own small 'Dragon' model. It was not long before he and a couple of friends invented computer games and was so full of his new life. He was still too young to leave at age 13, though. I just could not do that to him.

I think my work was beginning to suffer. I was not always as patient as I should have been. There were patients I was not particularly fond of, but usually hid it well enough, but lately I had let one or two get under my skin.

Molly Simpkins was referred for assessment and treatment of a leg ulcer. She had specifically asked me to arrive around ten in the morning, so I found myself at that time, driving down the muddy track to the old farmhouse nestled in a pretty bush-clad valley. I tried where possible to fit in with patient's requests as I know it was a frustration to await all day for a visit from the nurse.

I knocked at the door and a voice shouted 'come in.' I was surprised to step directly into the kitchen where four men were sitting round the large table. It was piled high with plates of steak, chops, sausages, and eggs. A mound of toast and thick mugs of tea and coffee were distributed among the ravenously eating men.

'Goodness, I am sorry; I didn't intend to interrupt your ... breakfast?'

'G'wan, this is our smoko. We've been on the go since five,' an older man who I took to be my patient's husband said through a shower of tea and crumbs as he bit into a huge slab of toast dripping with butter. He gestured with a grubby thumb to a woman sitting in the corner with her leg up on a stool, 'that's 'er.'

I edged round the table and spoke to the over-large lady wedged into an old armchair. Her grey hair was unkempt, and she had a dirty apron pinned with safety pins.

'Hello, Mrs Simpkins, I've come to do your leg. Would you like to go somewhere else for the dressing?' I looked over at the eating men, thinking that this was perhaps not the best place to be treating a leg ulcer.

'No, s'alright. I don't mind. He can have a good look at what I 'ave to put up with, 'e can.' I refrained from saying that it might put him off his food, as I suspected that it would not, and unwrapped the dressing. It was not the worst I had seen but certainly would have put me off a meal.

'Ere, Fred, come and look at this.' He got up, toast still in his hand and walked over; peered at his wife's leg, sniffed, and wandered back to the table without a word.

I attended to the cleaning, dressing and bandaging, trying to ignore the eating noises behind me and made a mental note to arrive a little later next visit.

Over the weeks I tried to time my visits to avoid the eating men, but often Molly Simpkins would phone and say it was not convenient to see me other than at ten in the morning. I learned to ignore the distractions, and gradually the ulcer started to heal, so that I did not have to call so often. I did not enjoy my visits. Mrs Simpkins was totally focused on her leg and the progress of the ulcer, insisting on her husband's monitoring it. She would peer at it intently and need to have assurance that it was altering shape and discuss at length the merits of various treatments. When I thought about my other patients waiting for my visits, some of whom were extremely ill, I resented the time Mrs Simpkins always tried to delay me.

At last, I was able to say, 'well, Mrs Simpkins, I think you can just put a small dry dressing and an elastic stocking on; it is about healed.' I saw she was upset and felt a little sorry for her. I then made a big mistake by saying, 'you can always give me a ring if you should have any trouble.'

It was only a week after I received a phone call from her; 'oh nurse, it's real bad again. Don't know what happened, can you call, say about ten this morning will do.'

I cursed under my breath and said she would have to wait as I had a terribly busy day. The thought of going back again annoyed me. 'What have you been doing? Picking at the scab? I told you just to put a dressing on and a bandage.'

It was a couple of days before I got round to visiting and when I did, I was horrified at what I found. The whole of Mrs Simpkins' lower leg was a mass of scratches and cuts, matted with blood and oozing pus.

'What on earth has happened?'

'I had to scratch and scratch. I need to have it looked after. No-one is interested anymore.'

I realised this was more than I could cope with and spoke to her doctor. Mrs Simpkins was admitted to hospital where she had all the attention she craved, but it left me feeling a little guilty. Perhaps if I had been more patient, accepting her problem was as much emotional as physical and kept visiting for longer, she would have avoided hospital.

4/15

One of the disadvantages with working on my own was the professional isolation. I was supposed to go to a meeting at our Headquarters each month but with increasing demand of visits I could rarely spare an afternoon. So it was with pleasure I sometimes had a student nurse or doctor drive around with me, to learn what happened when the patients arrived back in their own homes. It always amused me to see the amazement on their faces when confronted with the less clinical conditions we had to deal with.

'But what about infection, Sister,' one doctor exclaimed as I removed yet another crop of sutures from Frank Gregson, having finally run him to ground in his workshop.

'Well, in this case it is miracle that I have actually managed to get to the sutures before they fuse into his skin,' I said as I whipped out the last stitch. 'You can see, I am wearing surgical gloves and the dressing pack is sterile. And in any case,' I added as I collected up the dressings and instruments, 'the bugs in people's homes are their own. The only infected wounds I have had come with my patients from hospital.'

I found some of the young doctors very condescending. Most were in their last year of training, and after their many years of study, thought they knew everything.

'You see,' I continued on this occasion, 'you have to look at the whole person. As you see them they are just "an appendicectomy" or "a cancer case". You must remember you are discharging them into a home environment, where situations are vastly different.' I was not sure if I had made any impression but hoped some of my words had taken root.

Once a month or so, I was asked to take a student nurse on my rounds for a few days and then ask them to write a report and I had to mark it. Some of the girls had requested the experience, but others had been told to do it as part of their training. The latter were sometimes hard work and obviously regarded this as a day's holiday, not showing any interest in what they regarded as an unimportant aspect of their profession. To them, their work began and ended on the hospital ward. I did my best to awaken an interest, reasoning that if they had some idea of the reality of the home environment, they would be more sympathetic on the wards. I had learned from my times of working in a hospital how some patients worried about how the family were coping at home, or about a loss of income. This could slow the healing process.

Sometimes there was a little too much "reality" for a young person to accept.

I had been referred to visit a new patient who was a known diabetic, by one of the doctors. 'He's complaining about one of his feet; it may be affected by his diabetes. Have a look nurse, and let me know what you think, will you?' We had several such referrals. It saved the doctor's time and made it easier on less ambulant patients.

The old man lived in an area which was difficult to get to off the Muriwai road. I had been down the short access road before, which led to three or four small houses perched on the sides of a bush-clad valley. To the uninitiated it seemed as if the driver was heading over the side of the valley from the road into space. Access was through a one-car width lane which was not easily visible from the road, surrounded as it was by vegetation. It was necessary to drive into the dark cavern and slowly downwards on the muddy lane, keeping close to the cliff on one side and away from the sheer drop on the other. As traffic was both ways, I always said a private prayer that no vehicle was coming the other direction.

The student with me had been particularly annoying on this occasion. She made no effort to hide her boredom, tapping her fingers on the armrest and asking no questions. Normally I would have warned my passenger about the scary descent, but I was tired of her attitude.

'Let's see if this interests you,' I muttered, as I changed down to bottom gear and shot through the opening. She gave a gratifying shriek and clung onto the side of her seat.

'Hope we don't meet anyone, I'm not good at backing,' I cheerfully remarked.

We found the patient's place, little more than a shack, and as I pushed open the door, we could hear a low humming. 'Mr Hoffman! district nurse,' I called and walked into the house, 'come on nurse,' as she hesitated by the door.

'In here; in the bedroom, nurse.'

As I walked in the darkened room, I realised what the humming was; bluebottles; there seemed to be hundreds of them.

'Doctor asked me to come and look at you, Mr Hoffman. This is a student nurse with me for today. Is it OK if she comes in too?' I asked as she sidled into the room.

'Sure; sure. It's me foot. No pain but it sort of tickles.'

I pulled the ragged curtain aside, and a cloud of bluebottles swirled around the room. I was not looking at them, but at Mr Hoffman's foot; it was covered in a moving white mat. I looked closer and realised the blackened big toe was infested with maggots. I heard the student nurse gasp.

I was not too happy, myself.

'Er, well Mr Hoffman, I think I had better clean this up a bit and then the doctor needs to see your toe.' I turned to the young nurse and felt a little sorry for her, she was looking very pale. Well, she had to learn. 'Get me a dressing pack out would you please, we'll have to pick these off and swab with peroxide, though of course they are doing a good job to debride the dead tissue.' She silently got out the pack, but as soon as I started to pick off the maggots, she started to gag. 'Outside please nurse, you can sit in the car if you like.'

I was quite a while removing the wriggling little maggots, calling to mind stories of casualties in the First World war sometimes having only this treatment to treat their wounds in the field hospitals. It might have been better to leave them to do their job, but I was pretty sure the poor man was going to lose his toe, if not his foot.

On the drive back, the young girl said, 'I had no idea things like that happened and that you have to deal with it on your own.' She shivered, 'Ugh, I don't know how you could do that!'

'Well, you have to. You can't call someone else to do it.' I smiled at her. 'Never mind, you won't have to do things like that on the safety of your ward.'

'It has made me think a bit. You really need to be a special sort of nurse to do this job, don't you?' she said thoughtfully, she had obviously been shaken out of her apathy. 'I thought it was all driving about and giving showers and cutting old guy's toenails.'

'Well, some of that, too. A lot of the time while we are doing mundane things, we are keeping an eye on how they are managing. People have their own problems, but don't always talk about it. Try and remember that in the hospital.'

It was a thoughtful and sober young nurse who returned to her flat and I was very interested to receive her 'write up' about the visit a few days later; she really had her eyes opened and I marked her work fairly.

I admitted I did enjoy teaching the young nurses, so when I was approached to take a Sister Tutor's course a few weeks later, I gave it some serious thought.

When I discussed this with Ken, he was far from happy.

'But Chris you will have to travel into Auckland during the week. What about Roy and me?'

'It will mean a higher salary ... I would have thought that would appeal to you Ken. After all we are living off what I earn, aren't we?

After some heated discussion, eventually I had to abandon the idea, which I thought a little unfair of Ken. I would have been home for the weekends, and now Roy was in high school he was becoming more independent.

I do not know what Ken's objection was unless he saw it as a step towards my independence and the beginning of our eventual separation.

Which as the years passed seemed more and more likely and came to that dramatic resolution in the telephone booth in London Heathrow Airport.

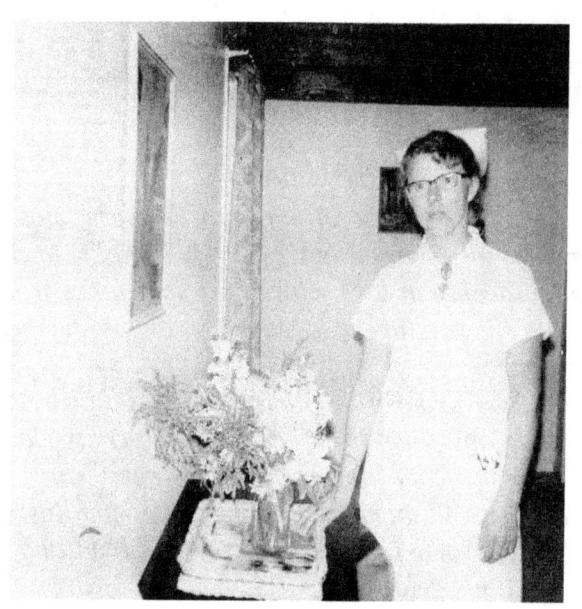

Chris at St Swithins

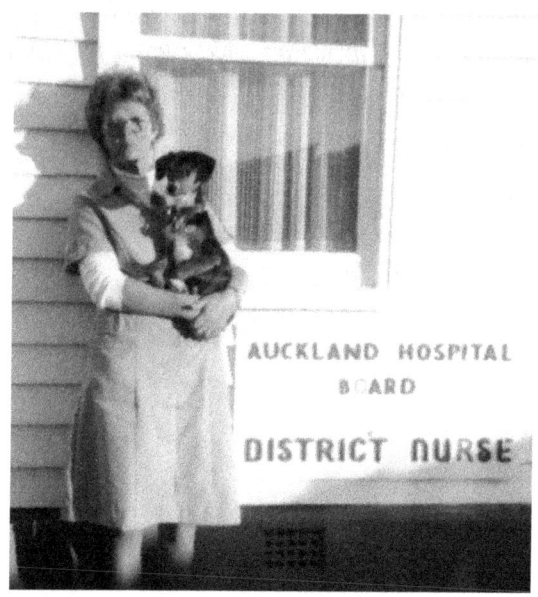

With Little dog Bitza

EPILOGUE

Neither of us realised circumstances were moving us forward to that eventual outcome. Had I not re-met Peter and fallen deeply in love with him I sometimes wonder if we would have stayed together, drawing further and further apart.

After our separation and eventual divorce, Ken married a long-time friend from our Scouts days and lived the rest of his life in the area where I had been a district nurse. We buried our differences for Roy's sake, visiting each other in Sark and New Zealand and stayed friends until his death.

For eight years I remained on Sark after the love of my life died, undecided what to do with the rest of my life. Financial pressures and Roy's return to New Zealand finally made my return there also inevitable.

After nearly forty-six years as a nurse, retirement was staring me in the face; what could I do now?

My answer was to take a creative writing course, where I discovered I had many tales to share with you my readers and I hope you can understand why when asked all those years ago 'So You want to be a nurse?' I answered; **Yes; Yes, Yes.**'

****